Certified Ophthalmic Assistant
Exam Study Guide

Executive Editor
Emanuel Newmark, MD, FACS

**AMERICAN ACADEMY
OF OPHTHALMOLOGY**
The Eye M.D. Association

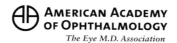
AMERICAN ACADEMY
OF OPHTHALMOLOGY
The Eye M.D. Association

The Academy provides this material for educational purposes only. It is not intended to represent the only or best method or procedure in every case, nor to replace a physician's own judgment or give specific advice for case management. Including all indications, contraindications, side effects, and alternative agents for each drug or treatment is beyond the scope of this material. All information and recommendations should be verified, prior to use, with current information included in the manufacturers' package inserts or other independent sources, and considered in light of the patient's condition and history. Reference to certain drugs, instruments, and other products in this publication is made for illustrative purposes only and is not intended to constitute an endorsement of such. Some materials may include information on applications that are not considered community standard, that reflect indications not included in approved FDA labeling, or that are approved for use only in restricted research settings. The FDA has stated that it is the responsibility of the physician to determine the FDA status of each drug or device he or she wishes to use, and to use them with appropriate patient consent in compliance with applicable law. The Academy specifically disclaims any and all liability for injury or other damages of any kind, from negligence or otherwise, for any and all claims that may arise out of the use of any recommendations or other information contained herein.

Financial Disclosures

The contributors disclose the following financial relationships. **Lama A. Al-Aswad, MD:** (S) Allergan, Congressional Glaucoma Caucus; (C, L, S) Alcon Laboratories. **Neil T. Choplin, MD:** (C) Carl Zeiss Meditec; (L) Alcon Laboratories, Allergen, Merck U.S. Human Health. **Mike P. Ehrenhaus, MD:** (C, L): Alcon Laboratories, Allergen, Inspire, Ista Pharmaceuticals. **Neil J. Friedman, MD:** (C, O): Optimedica, Oraya; (L) Alcon Laboratories, Allergan, Inspire. **Damien M. Goldberg, MD:** (L) Allergen, Inspire. **David Goldman, MD:** (C) Alcon Laboratories, Allergen. **Andrew A. Moshfeghi, MD:** (C) Alcon Laboratories, Optos; (C, L, S) Genentech. **Silvia Orengo-Nania, MD:** (C) Allergen; (C, L, S) Alcon Laboratories, Pfizer Ophthalmics. **Stephen R. Russell, MD:** (S) Alcon Laboratories. **Diana J. Shamis, MHSE, CO, COMT:** (L) SECO International, LLC.

The following contributors state that they have no significant financial interest or other relationship with the manufacturer of any commercial product discussed in their contributions to this module or with the manufacturer of any competing commercial product: Ann E. Bidwell, MD; Lee R. Duffner, MD, FACS; Joel M. Engelstein, MD; Erich P. Horn, MD; Kenneth B. Mitchell, MD; Emanuel Newmark, MD, FACS; Steven M. Shields, MD, FACS; George A. Stern, MD; Jay S. Wallshein, MD, MA.

C = Consultant fee, paid advisory boards or fees for attending a meeting
L = Lecture fees (honoraria), travel fees, or reimbursements when speaking at the invitation of a commercial entity
O = Equity ownership/stock options of publicly or privately traded firms (excluding mutual funds)
P = Patents and/or royalties that might be viewed as creating a potential conflict of interest
S = Grant support

Library of Congress Cataloging-in-Publication Data

Certified ophthalmic assistant exam study guide/executive editor, Emanuel Newmark; authors, Lama Al-Aswad ... [et al.].
    p. ; cm.
    Includes bibliographical references and index.
    ISBN 978-1-61525-100-1 (pbk. : alk. paper)
    1. Ophthalmic assistants–Examinations, questions, etc. 2. Ophthalmology–Examination Questions. I. Newmark, Emanuel, 1936–II. Al-Aswad, Lama. III. American Academy of Ophthalmology.
    [DNLM: 1. Ophthalmology–Examination Questions. 2. Ophthalmic Assistants–Examination Questions. WW 18.2 C418 2010]
    RE72.5.C47 2010
    617.70076–dc22
                                         2009052800

Printed in the United States of America
14 13 12 11 10   1 2 3 4

Authors

Emanuel Newmark, MD, FACS
Executive Editor
Atlantis, Florida

Lama A. Al-Aswad, MD
New York, New York

Ann E. Bidwell, MD
Chicago, Illinois

Neil T. Choplin, MD
San Diego, California

Lee R. Duffner, MD, FACS
Golden Beach, Florida

Mike P. Ehrenhaus, MD
Bayside, New York

Joel M. Engelstein, MD
Silver Spring, Maryland

Neil J. Friedman, MD
Palo Alto, California

Damien F. Goldberg, MD
Torrance, California

David A. Goldman, MD
Palm Beach Gardens, Florida

Erich P. Horn, MD
Oakland, California

Kenneth B. Mitchell, MD
Morgantown, West Virginia

Andrew A. Moshfeghi, MD, MBA
Palm Beach Gardens, Florida

Silvia D. Orengo-Nania, MD
Houston, Texas

Stephen R. Russell, MD
Iowa City, Iowa

Diana J. Shamis, MHSE, CO, COMT
Gainesville, Florida

Steven M. Shields, MD, FACS
Chesterfield, Missouri

George A. Stern, MD
Missoula, Montana

Jay S. Wallshein, MD, MA
Atlantis, Florida

Contents

Preface

Becoming a certified allied health professional in ophthalmology necessitates formal training, work experience, and passing the certified ophthalmic assistant (COA) examination, administered by the Joint Commission on Allied Health Personnel in Ophthalmology (JCAHPO). According to the United States Department of Labor, which now recognizes ophthalmic medical assisting as a specialized occupation, "Employers prefer to hire experienced workers or those who are certified. Although not required, certification indicates that a medical assistant meets certain standards of competence."

This book was conceived in response to feedback from readers of *Ophthalmic Medical Assisting: An Independent Course*, Fourth Edition, published by the Academy. This feedback indicated that readers wanted additional material to supplement *Ophthalmic Medical Assisting*: (1) content organized by the specific areas of knowledge tested by the COA exam; (2) a way to assess their own level of knowledge, so they would know which subject areas needed more attention; and (3) a practice test to simulate COA exam conditions.

The authors and I have worked hard to achieve these objectives. As further enhancements, many questions contain illustrations to add a visual component to learning, and all questions are accompanied not only by the answer but also an explanation for why that answer is correct and the alternatives are incorrect. We feel grateful to have participated in this project and confident we have succeeded in meeting our primary goal: to help ophthalmic medical assistants prepare for an important milestone of their careers.

Acknowledgments

I sincerely thank the contributors to this study guide, whose names appear elsewhere. These very busy individuals have taken time away from their practices, families, and leisure to create the content and review numerous sets of proofs. I am blessed to have had their cooperation, friendship, and dedication throughout this project. The Academy's Ophthalmology Liaison Committee provided guidance for the entire undertaking, including review of the content for scientific accuracy, and I thank them for their contributions.

I am exceedingly grateful for the hard work and generosity of the Academy's editorial staff and the Academy Board for approving this new publication. I am honored to have been asked to be its executive editor. I could not have accomplished this endeavor without the support of my wife, Tina. Having a Masters Degree in Health Education enabled her to provide valuable counsel and editorial assistance.

Lastly, I want to thank ophthalmic medical assistants for their desire to become certified and thereby sparking the creation of this publication. This study guide is dedicated to them, as well as my ophthalmologist colleagues who appreciate competent personnel and quality eye care.

Emanuel Newmark, MD, FACS
Executive Editor

Getting Started

The *Certified Ophthalmic Assistant Exam Study Guide* is organized into 4 sections:

- Section One, Self-Assessment, consists of 345 multiple-choice questions. It is organized into 19 subject areas (see below) and is intended to help you broadly assess your knowledge in each subject area. This section offers a review environment to study as your schedule allows. To start, pull out or copy the blank Answer Sheet at the end of Section One. Complete this section in your own time.
- Section Two, Self-Assessment Answers and Explanations, repeats the Section One questions, provides the correct answer, and explains why that answer is correct. You can compare your responses on the Answer Sheet to the Answer Key at the end of Section Two.
- Section Three, Practice Test, includes 100 different multiple-choice questions. The mix of questions is distributed across 19 subject areas in no particular order, to simulate the experience of taking the COA exam. As with the Self-Assessment section, you can pull out or copy the Answer Sheet and complete it. The 100-item test in this section should take no longer than 90 minutes to complete. Using a stopwatch or alarm clock when taking the Practice Test is very helpful.
- Section Four, Practice Test Answers and Explanations, repeats the Practice Test items in Section Three, provides the correct answer, and explains why that answer is correct. You can compare your answers to the Answer Key at the end of Section Four.

The Certified Ophthalmic Assistant

The Joint Commission on Allied Health Personnel in Ophthalmology (JCAHPO) is a nonprofit organization that offers certification and continuing education opportunities to ophthalmic allied health personnel. JCAHPO recognizes 3 official levels of certified ophthalmic medical personnel: *certified ophthalmic assistant* (COA), *certified ophthalmic technician* (COT), and *certified ophthalmic medical technologist* (COMT). JCAHPO certification attests to the skills and knowledge of individuals at each of these levels after they meet certain educational and experiential prerequisites and pass an examination. This credential provides evidence to employers and patients that the certified individual has achieved competence at the specified level. The JCAHPO credential is similar to the certification received by physicians or nurses who have met the requirements of their respective certification processes.

The Core Areas of Knowledge

The self-assessment modules in this Study Guide are organized into subject areas intended to mirror JCAHPO's content model for the COA exam.

These 19 subject areas include the following:

1. History Taking
2. Pupillary Assessment
3. Equipment Maintenance and Repair
4. Lensometry
5. Keratometry

6. Medical Ethics, Legal, and Regulatory Issues
7. Microbiology
8. Pharmacology
9. Ocular Motility
10. In-Office Minor Surgical Procedures
11. Ophthalmic Patient Services and Education
12. Ophthalmic Imaging
13. Refractometry
14. Spectacle Skills
15. Supplemental Skills
16. Tonometry
17. Visual Assessment
18. Visual Fields
19. Surgical Assisting in ASC or Hospital-Based OR

Note: The Academy does not warrant that the content of this guide actually reflects the official JCAHPO exam content or is the core knowledge that will be actually found on the examination. This guide, however, does contain important and practical information necessary for anyone employed as an ophthalmic medical assistant.

Study Tips

- This book can be used as a study tool for the COA exam, both for certification and recertification, or as a convenient, effective way to increase your knowledge and gain valuable feedback.
- In Sections Three and Four, each explanation of the correct answer includes, in parentheses, a short form of the source(s) for a particular question. For example, "Newmark 2006, 114, 220" is a short form of "Newmark E, ed. *Ophthalmic Medical Assisting: An Independent Study Course*, 4th ed. San Francisco: American Academy of Ophthalmology; 2006, 114, 220. Suggested Reading on page 253 has the full listing of the books, journals, and Web articles considered in the preparation of this book.

Most of the questions in this book use positive wording; ie, they emphasize best practice or the application of knowledge. In questions with a negative construction (for example, questions that include "no," "not," or "except") the negative words are printed in boldface. You may encounter this type of question in your test-taking experiences. Because a question with a negative construction can be more difficult to comprehend, these constructions are grouped together at the end of each content category.

Certified Ophthalmic Assistant Exam Study Guide Online

An online version of the *Certified Ophthalmic Assistant Exam Study Guide* is available for purchase from the Academy (www.aao.org). This online resource includes a self-study area in which you can browse the full database of questions that appear in this book. In addition, you may mark questions to revisit; see a summary of answered, unanswered, marked, and skipped questions prior to scoring; and bookmark, highlight, and add notes to questions for future reference. There are also 10 timed practice exams, using content from the Self-study area. The JCAHPO COA certification exam is a 3-hour, timed, online examination consisting of 200 questions. Each timed practice exam in the online product simulates an online exam experience, with 90 minutes to complete each 100-question module.

Additional Resources

The American Academy of Ophthalmology is the membership organization representing the vast majority of ophthalmologists in the United States and Canada. As part of its focus on clinical education, the Academy offers resources for ophthalmic medical personnel, such as this guide and other products described on the Academy Web site (www.aao.org). There are many other resources that publish information about or provide continuing education opportunities for ophthalmic personnel. Visit their Web sites for the latest information:

- American Orthoptic Council: www.orthoptics.org
- American Society of Ocularists: www.ocularist.org
- American Society of Ophthalmic Registered Nurses: www.asorn.org
- Association of Technical Personnel in Ophthalmology: www.atpo.org
- Contact Lens Association of Ophthalmologists: www.clao.org
- Contact Lens Society of America: www.clsa.info
- Ophthalmic Photographers Society: www.opsnet.org
- Opticians Association of America: www.oaa.org

Self-Assessment Modules

1 | HISTORY TAKING

1   Which of the following is part of a comprehensive medical history?

   a. past ocular history
   b. pachymetry
   c. biomicroscopy
   d. IOL calculation

2   What is the definition of a chief complaint?

   a. the condition causing the visual problem
   b. the condition explaining the patient's complaint
   c. the reason causing the patient to seek care
   d. a serious medical problem from the patient's past medical history

3   In what way should a patient's chief complaint be documented?

   a. in the patient's own words
   b. in the doctor's own words
   c. in the technician's own words
   d. in the patient's spouse's own words

4   If the patient comes to the exam room with a family member, how should the medical assistant proceed?

   a. Take a history from the family member.
   b. Ask the patient if the family member should be present for the visit.
   c. Ignore the family member.
   d. Ask the family member to leave the room.

5   If a small child is brought for a first exam by her mother (Mary Jones), what is the best way to address the patient's mother?

   a. "Mom, what is the reason for today's visit?"
   b. "Mary, what is the reason for today's visit?"
   c. "Ms. Jones, what is the reason for today's visit?"
   d. "Lady, what is the reason for today's visit?"

6   Why is it important to specifically inquire about a patient's occupational and recreational activities?

   a. It may identify mutually enjoyable activities, such as hiking or golf.
   b. Patients may be engaging in activities that are dangerous without proper ocular protection.
   c. Patients enjoy providing personal details about their lives.
   d. These questions distract patients from long waits to see the doctor.

7   When a history of sexually transmitted disease or illegal drug use is obtained, what is the next recommended step?

   a. Write this information in the chart in red pen.
   b. Write this information on a separate piece of paper.
   c. Talk with co-workers about the patient's history.
   d. Omit this information from the patient's record entirely.

8   While striking a metal bolt with a hammer, a patient developed severe pain after he felt something hit his eye. What type of injury would this most likely represent?

   a. chemical injury
   b. thermal injury
   c. penetrating injury
   d. toxin injury

2 | PUPILLARY ASSESSMENT

1   Which of the following medications will have an effect on pupil size or reactivity?
   a. tropicamide eyedrops
   b. ciprofloxacin eyedrops
   c. artificial tears
   d. proparacaine eyedrops

2   Examining the pupillary reactions can help locate abnormalities in which of the following?
   a. lens
   b. optic nerve
   c. extraocular muscles
   d. conjunctiva

3   When a light is shined into an eye, it is expected to cause the pupil on that side to constrict. Which reaction of the pupil does this test assess?
   a. direct reaction
   b. consensual reaction

c. delayed reaction

d. confrontational reaction

4 The pupil of a patient's eye constricts when the other eye is illuminated but fails to constrict when it is illuminated directly. This is an example of which defect?

a. consensual reaction defect

b. paradoxical reaction defect

c. reverse pupillary defect

d. afferent pupillary defect

5 Once pupils are dilated for a retinal exam, what can be stated about the pupillary reactions?

a. They are no longer reliable.

b. They should be easier to test.

c. They indicate intracranial pathology.

d. They may suggest drug abuse.

6 The size of the pupil may be measured easily using which method?

a. laser interferometer

b. magnetic resonance imaging (MRI)

c. computed tomography (CT)

d. ruler or gauge

7 An asymptomatic patient has been referred to the ophthalmologist for evaluation of anisocoria, or unequal pupil size. The examination confirms the finding that the right pupil is 1 mm larger than the left pupil, although both pupils show a normal direct response to light. What is the best next step to evaluate pupil function?

a. Test for consensual response of each pupil.

b. Use tropicamide drops to dilate each eye.

c. Use timolol maleate drops to constrict each pupil.

d. Test for paradoxical response of each pupil.

8 A pupillary examination can evaluate which of the following?

a. nerve damage

b. glaucoma

c. cataract

d. scleral disease

9 A light is shined into a patient's eye and the pupil of the other eye constricts. This is an example of which reaction?

a. direct reaction

b. paradoxical reaction

    c. confrontational reaction

    d. consensual reaction

10 During an examination of a new patient, an irregularly shaped pupil in one eye is noted. What is the best next course of action for the ophthalmic medical assistant?

    a. Dilate the patient's pupils.

    b. Discuss the findings with an ophthalmologist.

    c. Request anterior segment photographs.

    d. Perform cycloplegic retinoscopy.

3   EQUIPMENT MAINTENANCE AND REPAIR

1 Which of the following is a responsibility of ophthalmic medical assistants?

    a. Maintain the equipment directly used by themselves.

    b. Maintain the specific instruments they used that day.

    c. Clean only the instruments they use personally.

    d. Be responsible for all ophthalmic equipment whether they used the equipment themselves or not.

2 Which statement applies to optical lenses used in the ophthalmic practice?

    a. To prevent scratches they should not be cleaned.

    b. They can be cleaned with gauze soaked with saline solution.

    c. They can be cleaned with approved cleaning fluid.

    d. They can be cleaned with soft, dry facial tissue.

— 55D lens

3 Which statement applies to the Hruby lens?

    a. It allows a binocular view of the central fundus.

    b. It allows magnification of the peripheral fundus.

    c. It can be left in the same position after use.

    d. It should be soaked in solution in between each use.

4 What range of hand-held, noncontact, funduscopic lenses is used in conjunction with the slit lamp?

    a. +20 D to +40 D

    b. +60 D to +90 D

    c. +40 D to +60 D

    d. +20 D to +50 D

5   If an electrical instrument fails to work, which of the following should be initiated first?

 a. Confirm that the instrument is plugged into the electric wall outlet.
 b. Call a licensed electrician.
 c. Change the fuse.
 d. Call the doctor to the room.

6   The phoropter is associated with which of the following features?

 a. It is used to perform a subjective lensometry.
 b. It is available only with nondisposable shields that need to be cleaned between uses.
 c. It should be cleaned front and back with alcohol and a soft, dry cloth.
 d. It should be scheduled for maintenance every 2 years.

7   If the slit-lamp light does not operate, what should the technician do?

 a. Check the electrical wall outlet plug and the instrument fuse and bulb.
 b. Check the internal transformer connections.
 c. Do not replace the bulb if it seems to be in good condition.
 d. Call the doctor to the room.

8   Which of the following instruments provides a stereoscopic view of the retina?

 a. direct ophthalmoscope
 b. retinoscope
 c. gonioscope
 d. head-mounted indirect ophthalmoscope

9   Care of the Snellen chart projector unit includes which of the following steps?

 a. Clean the slides with warm water or cleansing solutions.
 b. Clean the viewing mirrors with lint-free cloth or compressed air.
 c. Wait until the bulb goes completely dark before replacing it.
 d. Clean the external lens surfaces and focusing tubes once every 2 years to ensure they are clear.

10   Which of the following statements applies to the tip of the Goldmann-type tonometer?

 a. The prism tip contacts the eye and flattens a small area of the sclera by a known pressure or force.
 b. The prism tip should be thoroughly cleaned with an alcohol sponge and allowed to air dry.
 c. The prism tip should be cleansed by soaking with 10% hydrogen peroxide or regular household bleach.
 d. The prism tip can be used immediately after soaking.

11   What is the proper way to care for a Tono-Pen?

   a. Clean the metal tip periodically of debris with compressed air.
   b. Clean the latex cover between each use.
   c. Store the unit without the tip covered.
   d. Replace the batteries whenever the readout displays "BAD."

12   Common types of ophthalmic lasers include which of the following?

   a. argyle
   b. kryptonian
   c. exciser
   d. neodymium:yttrium-aluminum garnet

13   The manual lensmeter unit includes an eyepiece, lens holder, light source, and adjustment knobs. Proper maintenance of the unit includes which step?

   a. Blow dust from the lens surfaces with a clean, dry bulb syringe or compressed air.
   b. Wipe the external enamel finish with a jeweler's polishing cloth to prevent buildup.
   c. Lubricate the instrument if it feels tight.
   d. Use lens cleanser or detergent to clean the lens surfaces.

14   Which statement is **incorrect** about the medical assistant's participation in the care of ophthalmic lenses and equipment?

   a. The medical assistant should calibrate the automated computerized perimeter on a daily basis.
   b. Basic care is the responsibility of the medical assistant.
   c. Items should remain clean and in good working condition in order to function reliably.
   d. The medical assistant should calibrate the laser instruments once yearly.

15   Guidelines for cleaning noncontact lenses and mirrored surfaces include all **except** which of the following?

   a. Remove debris from lenses with an approved liquid by rubbing them with a lint-free cleaning cloth.
   b. Rub the lenses in a circular fashion to remove oils and fingerprints.
   c. Clean the lens at the first signs of dirt or debris.
   d. Thoroughly clean the optical mirrors with a dry lint-free cloth.

16   Guidelines for care of electrically powered instruments include all **except** which of the following?

   a. Cover instruments with a dust cover when not in use.
   b. Turn off everything in the exam rooms when not in use, except instruments being re-charged.
   c. Unplug equipment when performing any servicing except changing bulbs.
   d. Handle all bulbs with lens tissue paper to prevent oils from etching the bulb once it heats up.

17 Which of the following lenses **does not** contact the eye?

    a. goniolens
    b. Koeppe lens
    c. 3-mirror fundus lens
    d. Hruby lens

18 What guideline does **not** apply for cleaning lenses that make contact with the eye?

    a. Rinse them thoroughly with lukewarm water to remove contaminants.
    b. After cleaning, blot them dry with a paper towel.
    c. Disinfect or sterilize them between use.
    d. Sterilize lenses that are used during surgery or on a recently operated eye.

19 Which of the following is **not** considered a feature of the retinoscope?

    a. It is a hand-held instrument.
    b. It consists of a light source and a recording component.
    c. It is often powered by battery or rechargeable power packs.
    d. It is cleaned by blowing dust off the front surface with a clean bulb syringe.

20 Regarding equipment maintenance and repair, which of the following is **not** performed by the ophthalmic medical assistant?

    a. cleaning lenses and equipment
    b. protecting instruments from dust and damage
    c. calibrating lasers
    d. replacing light bulbs and fuses

4 LENSOMETRY

1 While checking progressive lens eyeglasses in a lensmeter, the technician notices that the lensmeter mires are centered on the third circle below the center of the lensmeter target by both lenses of the eyeglasses. What does this indicate?

    a. The progressive lenses are in the lensmeter upside down.
    b. There is base-down prism in both lenses of the eyeglasses.
    c. The lensmeter is out of alignment.
    d. The eyeglasses should be turned around to read the power from the other surface of the eyeglass lenses.

2 When looking through the eyepiece of a lensmeter, if the single line focuses at −4.00 D and the triple lines focus at −1.25D, what is the cylinder power?

    a. −6.25 D
    b. +2.75 D

   c. +3.20 D
   d. −2.75 D

3   Which of the following is the correct order for a written eyeglass prescription?

   a. sphere power, cylinder power, sphere axis
   b. sphere power, cylinder axis, cylinder power
   c. sphere power, cylinder power, cylinder axis
   d. sphere power, sphere axis, cylinder power

4   Neutralizing optical lenses is accomplished by which process?

   a. refractometry
   b. lensometry
   c. retinoscopy
   d. pachymetry

5   What is the first step in determining the prescription of a pair of eyeglasses with the lensmeter?

   a. Clean the lenses before reading.
   b. Adjust the eyepiece of the instrument.
   c. Position the frame on the spectacle table with the temples away from you.
   d. Turn the power drum to focus the mires to zero.

6   What statement about lensmeter measurement of prisms is true?

   a. It measures the power and orientation of the prism base.
   b. It measures only base up and base in prism.
   c. It measures only base down and base out prism.
   d. It measures the power and axis of the prism.

7   What statement is true about the optical center of a lens?

   a. The optical center of a lens is placed at the lower eyelid margin.
   b. The optical center of a lens is placed directly in front of the pupil.
   c. Lenses that are not optically centered can result in an off-axis prescription.
   d. The Geneva lens clock can determine the optical center of a lens.

8   The lensmeter reads the distance portion of a lens prescription to be −1.50 sphere. When reading the bifocal add, the lensmeter drum reads +1.25. What is the strength of the bifocal add in this prescription?

   a. +1.25
   b. +1.00
   c. +2.75
   d. +2.00

9   What is true about the intermediate segment in a trifocal lens?

    a. It is always half the power of the bifocal.
    b. It can be read with the PAL reader.
    c. It can be read using the lensmeter.
    d. It is twice the power of the bifocal add.

10   The following occurs while taking a lensmeter reading: the single lines focus at −3.00; the triple lines focus at −4.50 with the axis at 055°. What would be the eyeglass prescription?

    a. −4.50 −3.00 axis 145
    b. −3.00 −4.50 axis 055
    c. −3.00 −2.50 axis 145
    d. −3.00 −1.50 axis 055

11   What maneuver should be performed before adjusting the eyepiece on the lensmeter to obtain the most accurate reading?

    a. Turn the eyepiece to reflect the axis of your astigmatism.
    b. Turn the eyepiece to the most minus position.
    c. Turn the eyepiece to the neutral position.
    d. Turn the eyepiece to the most plus position.

12   During lensometry, what is the prism power and orientation of a right lens where the focused lines are displaced to the right and the lines cross at the second circle?

    a. 4 prism diopters base down
    b. 2 prism diopters base out
    c. 2 prism diopters base in
    d. 4 prism diopters base up

5 | KERATOMETRY

1   What is the method used to measure astigmatism?

    a. A-scan ultrasound
    b. ocular coherence tomography
    c. lensometry
    d. keratometry

2   What is the first step in performing manual keratometry?

    a. Center the reticule in the bottom right circle.
    b. Focus the cross hairs.
    c. Align the axes.
    d. Fuse the plus signs and the minus signs.

3   What is an important step in performing keratometry?

    a. Occlude the eye not being measured.
    b. Keep both eyes looking through the machine.
    c. Occlude the eye being tested.
    d. Put the correct prism in the device for accurate measurements.

4   The manual keratometer measures how much of the cornea?

    a. the whole corneal curvature
    b. approximately 3 mm of the center
    c. approximately 8 mm of the center
    d. the periphery and the center separately

5   What is the average corneal curvature of the human eye?

    a. 39.00 D
    b. 41.00 D
    c. 43.00 D
    d. 45.00 D

6   When the keratometer is properly aimed at the eye, how many circles will you see?

    a. 1 circle
    b. 2 circles
    c. 3 circles
    d. 4 circles

7   Keratometry is useful for which of the following?

    a. measuring the dioptric power of the cornea
    b. determining the power of glasses
    c. measuring the length of the eye
    d. determining the health of the retina

8   What is the way to find the proper axis in keratometry?

    a. Rotate the keratometer until a plus and minus sign align.
    b. Dial the vertical scale knob until the reflection in the keratometer is greatest.
    c. Rotate the keratometer until the 2 plus signs align.
    d. Rotate the horizontal scale knob until the reflection is dimmest.

9   Which of the following applies to keratometry in the fitting of contact lenses?

    a. not useful because the fit is based on the power of the lens
    b. useful because a good fit depends on corneal curvature
    c. should be used only in hard contact lens fittings
    d. does not work well when fitting soft lenses because it is too inaccurate

10   Why is keratometry helpful in fitting contact lenses?

a. because the axis of the astigmatism is all that is needed
b. because it measures all of the parameters needed to fit a contact lens
c. because it measures the astigmatism to fit toric contact lenses exclusively
d. because a good fit requires both the axis and the amount of astigmatism

6 | MEDICAL ETHICS, LEGAL, AND REGULATORY ISSUES

1   One of the medical principals of ethics is that physicians should practice medicine primarily for the benefit of the patient. What is the primary responsibility of the ophthalmic medical assistant?

a. to work primarily for the benefit of the patient
b. to abide by state medical laws
c. to perform all tasks requested in an emergency
d. to treat the patient with respect, as the patient is always right

2   Ethics are moral principles and values that govern individual behavior. Which of the following statements best applies to the professional code of ethics of the American Academy of Ophthalmology?

a. The Code broadens the perspective of assistants.
b. The Code requires physicians to set similar fees.
c. The Code requires physicians to answer all patients' questions.
d. The Code applies to all personnel on a member's staff.

3   Which governing body recognizes JCAHPO certification and why?

a. Federal and state governments recognize JCAHPO certification as part of hospital or clinic licensing requirements.
b. The American Board of Specialty Boards recognizes JCAHPO certification to ensure oversight of medical assistants.
c. Employers recognize JCAHPO certification as evidence of having achieved a certain level of competence.
d. Some state medical boards recognize JCAHPO certification as sufficient for diagnosis but not treatment of some eye conditions.

4   What does HIPAA protect?

a. patient's privacy
b. patient's finances
c. patient's ability to decide the course of treatment
d. patient's right for a second opinion

5   Under HIPAA (Health Insurance Portability and Accountability Act) regulations, the doctor may without permission disclose medical information to which of the patient's relationships?

a. spouse
b. child
c. physician(s)
d. attorney

6   Mrs. Smith's daughter calls the office to discuss her mother's medical condition. What should you do?

a. Give her all the information she asked for.
b. Ask for approval from Mrs. Smith to discuss her medical condition with her daughter.
c. Do not discuss it but give her a copy of the record.
d. Give her the diagnosis but no other information.

7   You saw your neighbor in the office last week. If you reveal her medical information to her friends without her permission, which of the following would apply?

a. You may be fined under state law.
b. You may be jailed under HIPAA law.
c. Your employer may be held responsible for a fine or criminal violation.
d. All of the above apply.

8   Why is informed consent important?

a. It is necessary to have so that the physician is protected.
b. It is necessary that the patient understands the procedure and its risks and benefits.
c. It is required by the hospital.
d. It is needed only for major surgery.

9   Which of the following best describes informed consent?

a. It is a signature on the permission form.
b. It is a protection for the surgeon.
c. It is a protection for the clinic.
d. It is a process.

10   In obtaining valid informed consent, which of the following factors must be considered?

a. native language of the patient
b. IQ of the patient
c. mood of the patient
d. prior surgical experiences of the patient

11   Which statement is correct regarding prescription medications?

a. Many prescriptions may be called in to the pharmacy by the ophthalmic medical assistant.
b. All prescriptions must include the doctor's license number.
c. Prescriptions to be filled as needed must be undated.
d. Only controlled substances such as narcotics require refill instructions.

12   Which of the following responses applies to unauthorized removal of drugs or eyedrops from a medical office or hospital?

a. This is allowed for temporary emergency treatment.
b. This is unlawful and unethical.
c. This is allowed to treat an indigent or self-pay patient.
d. This triggers an investigation by the Drug Enforcement Administration (DEA).

13   If during history taking you suspect domestic abuse, what should you do?

a. Call 911 or the local domestic abuse hotline.
b. Talk to the ophthalmologist immediately.
c. Document your interpretation in the medical record.
d. Order x-rays to document hidden or old fractures.

14   If you are the first person to discover a fallen patient, what should you do?

a. Assist the patient into a chair.
b. Arrange for the patient's transportation to the emergency room.
c. Start CPR.
d. Notify the physician.

15   The Centers for Disease Control (CDC) developed universal precautions to reduce transmission of which of the following?

a. viruses (such as HIV)
b. bacteria (such as methicillin-resistant *Staphylococcus aureus*)
c. parasites (such as toxoplasmosis)
d. prions (such as mad-cow disease)

16   The Centers for Disease Control (CDC) has designated "body substance isolation precautions." Regarding these precautions, which of the following statements applies?

a. They are mandated by OSHA (Occupational Safety & Health Administration).
b. They are not included in "standard precautions."
c. They apply to excimer laser exposure.
d. They do not apply to tears, aqueous, and vitreous if uncontaminated by blood.

17   Which of the following statements applies to universal precautions and hand washing?

    a. Hand washing is not required before wearing gloves.
    b. Hand washing is not required after wearing gloves.
    c. Hand washing with a germicide sterilizes the skin.
    d. Hand washing is required by OSHA.

18   Increasingly specific diagnoses can be coded using the ICD-9-CM system (International Classification of Diseases, ninth revision, clinical modification) by adding additional digits to a more general diagnosis code. Which of the following statements best characterizes ICD-9-CM coding?

    a. When a diagnosis is not known, no ICD-9-CM code should be applied.
    b. When a diagnosis is not known, a suspected diagnosis should be applied.
    c. Coding should be finalized to the highest level of specificity.
    d. A diagnosis cannot be a symptom.

19   Which of the following statements applies to medical coding?

    a. Coding is the language of processing insurance claims.
    b. Coding is acceptable as documentation for service provided.
    c. Coding makes no distinction between diagnoses and procedures.
    d. Coding facilitates understanding of disease complexity.

20   Ophthalmic medical assistants are not allowed to practice independently of a physician; however, they may always perform which of the following?

    a. Diagnose a condition.
    b. Suggest a treatment.
    c. Estimate a prognosis.
    d. Provide an explanation of why and how a test will be performed.

21   Which of the following is **not** part of a proper informed consent?

    a. discussion of the disease or problem for which surgery is proposed
    b. an agreement not to sue the doctor
    c. discussion of the risks and benefits of the proposed surgery
    d. discussion of alternative treatments

7 MICROBIOLOGY

1   Which of the following is a bacterium?

    a. herpes
    b. *Streptococcus*

      c. *Histoplasma*
      d. *Acanthamoeba*

2   Contact lens wearers who use homemade solution to clean their lenses are most likely to develop a corneal infection caused by which type of organism?

      a. bacteria
      b. virus
      c. fungi
      d. protozoa

3   What is the organism that is often associated with improper contact lens wear?

      a. *Staphylococcus aureus*
      b. *Pseudomonas aeruginosa*
      c. *Bacillus cereus*
      d. *Neisseria gonorrhoeae*

4   Which statement is correct regarding ocular infections?

      a. Herpes simplex virus types I and II may cause ocular infections.
      b. Protozoa that cause ocular infections have very limited distribution in the environment.
      c. Treatment of fungal infections is shorter in duration and less difficult than treatment of bacterial infections.
      d. Varicella-zoster virus and adenovirus infections cause shingles.

5   Which statement is correct regarding infection control precautions?

      a. Blood-soaked gauze should be placed in a rigid, puncture-proof biohazard container.
      b. Use of gloves to avoid contact with blood or body fluids makes hand washing unnecessary.
      c. Hand washing is one of the most important of the standard precautions.
      d. Universal precautions are used if blood has tested positive for pathogens.

6   Which statement is correct regarding disinfection?

      a. Disinfection may be accomplished with application of heat or chemicals.
      b. Disinfection takes longer than sterilization but more completely kills disease-causing microorganisms.
      c. Tonometer tips require no further disinfection if allowed to dry between patients.
      d. Cleaning equipment to remove organic material is not required if disinfection is performed immediately after use.

8 | PHARMACOLOGY

1   Which statement is correct regarding topical eye medication?

    a. Suspensions do not require a preservative.
    b. Solutions prevent systemic absorption.
    c. Properly administered ointments do not blur vision.
    d. Suspensions must be shaken vigorously before use.

2   The term *subcutaneous* refers to an injection that is given in what location?

    a. into the eye
    b. into a vein
    c. into a muscle
    d. under the skin

3   What is the act of dilating the pupil called?

    a. mydriasis
    b. cycloplegia
    c. pupilloplasty
    d. miosis

4   When is dapiprazole 0.5% ophthalmic solution used?

    a. to dilate the pupil
    b. to reverse pupillary dilation
    c. to treat infection
    d. to reduce inflammation

5   When administering a drop to a patient, where should the technician instruct the patient to look?

    a. Look up with the head tilted forward.
    b. Look up with the head tilted backward.
    c. Look down with the head tilted forward.
    d. Look down with the head tilted backward.

6   Which statement is correct regarding side effects of ophthalmic medications?

    a. Miotics may cause rapid pulse and dry mouth.
    b. Anesthetics prevent an allergic reaction by deadening a nerve.
    c. Cycloplegics may precipitate an attack of angle-closure glaucoma.
    d. Unlike systemic corticosteroid therapy, topical application does not cause cataracts.

7   An ophthalmic assistant accidentally instills a drop of atropine 1% instead of tropicamide (Mydriacyl 1%) into a patient's eyes. What should the assistant do immediately?

   a. Inform the patient that he will require sunglasses for 2 weeks.
   b. Inform the patient that his eyes will be dilated for 2 weeks.
   c. Inform the ophthalmologist.
   d. Rinse the cul-de-sac with sterile saline.

8   Which of the following medications may cause rapid pulse?

   a. atropine
   b. timolol
   c. nepafenac
   d. neomycin

9   Which statement is correct regarding ophthalmic medications?

   a. All cycloplegic eyedrops may cause stinging when administered topically.
   b. Suspensions remain on the ocular surface longer than solutions by preventing nasolacrimal drainage.
   c. Local injection of anesthetics prevents systemic toxicity.
   d. Unlike administration by injection, ophthalmic dyes administered topically do not cause allergic reactions.

10   Before Goldmann applanation tonometry is performed, it is most appropriate to instill which type of eyedrop?

   a. anesthetic
   b. antimicrobial
   c. cycloplegic
   d. miotic

11   In a healthy eye, fluorescein dye should cause fluorescence (a bright yellow-green color under cobalt blue lighting) only of which one of the following?

   a. tear film
   b. conjunctiva
   c. cornea
   d. iris

12   What dye is injected intravenously before angiography to highlight the retinal vessels?

   a. lissamine green
   b. fluorescein
   c. rose bengal
   d. gentian violet

13   Which of the following is an anesthetic?

    a. proparacaine (Alcaine)
    b. pilocarpine (Isopto-Carpine)
    c. travoprost (Travatan)
    d. mannitol (Osmitrol)

14   Brow ache, myopia, and retinal detachment are possible side effects of what type of medication?

    a. miotics
    b. cycloplegics
    c. carbonic anhydrase inhibitors
    d. prostaglandin analogs

15   If a patient reports a history of severe allergy to fluoroquinolones, what ophthalmic medicine might be dangerous for the patient?

    a. tobramycin drops
    b. ciprofloxacin drops
    c. timolol maleate drops
    d. acetazolamide tablets

16   Which statement is correct regarding antimicrobial therapy?

    a. So-called "fortified" antibiotics are available without a prescription.
    b. Topical antibiotics inhibit bacterial growth but systemic antibiotics kill bacteria.
    c. Single antifungal or antiviral agents are widely used as a preventive measure.
    d. Antivirals inhibit the ability of viruses to reproduce.

17   A patient has a flare-up of iritis. What is the most appropriate topical medication for treating this problem?

    a. proparacaine ophthalmic solution
    b. cyclosporine A emulsion
    c. prednisolone acetate 1% suspension
    d. timolol 1% solution

18   Corticosteroids can cause which of the following?

    a. cataract
    b. lower intraocular pressure
    c. encourage faster healing
    d. increase growth of eye muscles

19   Cyclosporine A (Restasis) is a topical emulsification used in the treatment of what condition?

    a. allergy
    b. uveitis
    c. tear deficiency
    d. glaucoma

20   Mast-cell stabilizers, such as cromolyn (Crolom), are useful in the treatment of which one of the following?

    a. bacterial infection
    b. seasonal allergic conjunctivitis
    c. intraocular inflammation
    d. glaucoma

21   If a medication is written to be taken prn, when should it be taken?

    a. before meals
    b. before bedtime
    c. with food
    d. as needed

22   If the doctor's prescription indicates the abbreviation qid, how often should the medication be administered?

    a. once a day
    b. every hour
    c. 4 times a day
    d. every 4 hours

23   The abbreviation tid refers to a medication that is to be administered how often?

    a. every 3 hours
    b. 3 times a day
    c. every 4 hours
    d. 4 times a day

24   Which of the following is an acute drug reaction?

    a. fainting
    b. headache
    c. salty taste in mouth
    d. sneezing

25   Medications that may impair the blood-clotting mechanism are important to know about before surgery. These medications include which of the following?

    a. aspirin
    b. acetaminophen
    c. morphine
    d. codeine

26   Which of the following statements is accurate?

    a. Topical decongestants remove the cause of ocular irritation.
    b. Topical and systemic corticosteroid therapies may cause glaucoma and cataracts.
    c. Mast-cell stabilizers maintain an appropriate tear film balance.
    d. Preservative-free lubricants do not cause side effects.

27   Decongestants such as Visine can cause all **except** which one of the following?

    a. allergy
    b. angle-closure glaucoma
    c. rebound redness
    d. elevated blood sugar

28   The principal uses of a cycloplegic agent include all **except** which of the following?

    a. performing a refraction that requires an absence of accommodation
    b. decreasing a ciliary muscle spasm present in patients with uveitis
    c. conducting a fundus examination
    d. treating open-angle glaucoma

29   Which injection type is **not** classified as systemic drug delivery?

    a. intravitreal injection
    b. intravenous injection
    c. intramuscular injection
    d. subcutaneous injection

30   Which of the following dye–color matches is **incorrect**?

    a. lissamine green – green
    b. rose bengal – rose
    c. fluorescein – yellow/green
    d. gentian violet – purple

31   Which of the following glaucoma medications is **not** a beta-adrenergic-blocker?

    a. timolol (Timoptic, Betimol)
    b. levobunolol (Betagan)
    c. mannitol (Osmitrol)
    d. carteolol (Ocupress)

32   Which of the following is **not** a nonsteroidal anti-inflammatory drug (NSAID)?

    a. diclofenac (Voltaren)
    b. flurbiprofen (Ocufen)
    c. loteprednol etabonate (Lotemax)
    d. bromfenac (Xibrom)

9 OCULAR MOTILITY

1   What is an outward deviation of the eye called?

    a. exo deviation
    b. eso deviation
    c. hyper deviation
    d. hypo deviation

2   What combination of extraocular muscle actions occur when a patient looks to her left?

    a. left lateral rectus contracts; right lateral rectus relaxes
    b. left lateral rectus contracts; right lateral rectus contracts
    c. left medial rectus contracts; right lateral rectus relaxes
    d. left medial rectus relaxes; right medial rectus relaxes

3   What is tested when the cardinal positions of gaze are evaluated?

    a. convergence
    b. divergence
    c. fusion
    d. function of the 6 extraocular muscles

4   When performing the cover-uncover test, the examiner notices that the uncovered eye moves in order to fix on the target. What does this probably represent?

    a. tropia
    b. suppression
    c. phoria
    d. amblyopia

5   The size of an ocular deviation may be measured by which of the following?

    a. prism and alternate cover test
    b. Worth 4-dot test
    c. Titmus fly
    d. exophthalmometer

6   During the cover-uncover test, neither eye moves when the cover is removed. This probably represents which of the following?

    a. tropia
    b. suppression
    c. orthophoria
    d. amblyopia

10 IN-OFFICE MINOR SURGICAL PROCEDURES

1   Prior to the patient's procedure, what is the assistant's major responsibility?

    a. Answer questions about the procedure.
    b. Put the patient at ease.
    c. Discuss the surgeon's ability to do the procedure.
    d. Discuss the disease process.

2   During minor office procedures, anesthesia often consists of which of the following?

    a. topical drops or locally injected anesthetic agents
    b. general inhalation anesthesia
    c. intravenous sedation
    d. tranquilizer

3   Which of the following is an instrument used to grasp tissue?

    a. scissors
    b. needle holder
    c. cannula
    d. forceps

4   What instrument is used to stop bleeding?

    a. forceps
    b. cannula
    c. clamp
    d. needle

5   What common minor surgical procedure is performed in the exam lane?

    a. cataract surgery
    b. ptosis repair
    c. trabeculectomy
    d. epilation

6   Which phrase applies to the insertion of punctual plugs?

  a. requires an anesthetic injection
  b. is a method of managing dry eyes
  c. is a cure for dry eyes
  d. is painful

7   Which of the following patients is a poor candidate for LASIK?

  a. a patient with myopic astigmatism
  b. a patient with hyperopic astigmatism
  c. a patient with a normal but thick cornea
  d. a patient with a normal but thin cornea

8   Which statement applies to refractive surgery?

  a. It is a minor procedure with minimal risks.
  b. It almost always results in the elimination of the need for glasses or contact lenses for the patient's lifetime.
  c. It is performed only with a laser.
  d. It often results in a decreased need for glasses or contact lenses.

9   What type of refractive *intraocular* surgery, although controversial, is currently being performed?

  a. LASIK and LASEK
  b. phakic intraocular lenses
  c. photorefractive Keratectomy (PRK)
  d. astigmatic Keratotomy (AK)

10   During a surgical procedure that does not involve general sedation, how can the assistant best help the surgeon?

  a. by remaining very quiet
  b. by talking to the patient for reassurance
  c. by anticipating the surgeon's next step
  d. by preparing the surgical site

11   An ophthalmologist usually performs surgery in all **except** which of the following sites?

  a. operating room
  b. office exam lanes
  c. minor operating room
  d. patient's home

12   Many minor surgical procedures can be performed in the ophthalmologist's office. They all have certain aspects in common **except** which of the following?

a. explaining the purpose of the procedure and obtaining the patient's consent
b. preparing the instruments and supplies
c. assisting the ophthalmologist during the procedure
d. having the patient call the ophthalmologist

13   The sterile operating field includes all **except** which of the following?

a. surgical gowns
b. instrument tray
c. protective eyewear
d. drapes

14   What instrument is **not** typically a part of a chalazion surgical set?

a. scalpel blade and handle
b. micro scissors
c. curette
d. needle holder

15   Which injection type is **not** classified as systemic drug delivery?

a. intravitreal injection
b. intravenous injection
c. intramuscular injection
d. subcutaneous injection

16   Which of the following items is **not** considered part of the sterile field?

a. the prepped part of the patient's body covered by a sterile drape
b. the tables and trays covered with a sterile drape and the sterile instruments
c. the surgical personnel, gowned and gloved
d. the chest, arms, and hands of the patient

11 OPHTHALMIC PATIENT SERVICES AND EDUCATION

1   In the following list, which is the best pairing?

a. optician: diagnosis of optical problems
b. ophthalmic assistant: removal of turned-in lashes
c. optometrist: LASIK surgery
d. ophthalmologist: informed consent process

2   What is a wedge-shaped growth of conjunctival tissue that grows onto the cornea?

    a. chalazion
    b. pinguecula
    c. nevus
    d. pterygium

3   What is the medical term for blood in the anterior chamber?

    a. rubeosis iridis
    b. hypopyon
    c. blunt trauma
    d. hyphema

4   What is the term for a turning in of the lower eyelid margin?

    a. ectropion
    b. ptosis
    c. trichiasis
    d. entropion

5   Which of the following is found in the conjunctiva?

    a. goblet cells
    b. meibomian glands
    c. lacrimal sac
    d. cilia

6   What is the condition referring to inflammation of the lacrimal sac?

    a. canaliculitis
    b. dacryoadenitis
    c. trichiasis
    d. dacryocystitis

7   The anterior chamber angle is formed by the junction of which structures?

    a. ciliary body and lens zonules
    b. cornea and sclera
    c. cornea and iris
    d. anterior and posterior chamber

8   Where are floaters found?

    a. aqueous humor
    b. lens
    c. vitreous
    d. retina

9   Through which structures does light pass before reaching the photoreceptors (rods and cones)?

   a. ganglion cells
   b. retinal pigment epithelium
   c. ciliary body
   d. choroid

10   Melanoma of the choroid is an example of what type of disease?

   a. infectious process
   b. degenerative process
   c. metabolic process
   d. neoplastic process

11   Multiple sclerosis (MS) is a chronic disease of the nervous system. It is often associated with what condition?

   a. exophthalmos
   b. scleritis
   c. intermittent droopy eyelids (ptosis)
   d. optic neuritis

12   Exophthalmos often occurs in which disease?

   a. rheumatoid arthritis
   b. Graves disease
   c. diabetes
   d. sarcoidosis

13   What is the correct *general* term when the eyes are not able to fixate on the same visual target due to a misalignment of the globes?

   a. diplopia
   b. exotropia
   c. strabismus
   d. amblyopia

14   Trichiasis is usually caused by which of the following disorders?

   a. entropion
   b. lagophthalmos
   c. blepharitis
   d. ptosis

15   Ophthalmia neonatorum refers to which condition in a newborn?

   a. conjunctivitis
   b. keratitis

    c. iritis

    d. retinopathy

16   A pinguecula is a degeneration of which ocular tissue?

    a. uvea

    b. sclera

    c. cornea

    d. conjunctiva

17   There are how many extraocular muscles?

    a. 4

    b. 5

    c. 6

    d. 7

18   What is the term for a layer of pus in the anterior chamber?

    a. rubeosis

    b. episcleritis

    c. hypopyon

    d. hyphema

19   The levator muscle attaches to what structure?

    a. tarsus

    b. orbicularis

    c. conjunctiva

    d. sclera

20   In primary angle-closure glaucoma, the aqueous outflow channel in the anterior chamber is blocked by which of the following?

    a. ciliary body

    b. cornea

    c. iris

    d. lens

21   Which statement is correct regarding open-angle glaucoma?

    a. It is more common earlier in life.

    b. It is more common in hyperopia.

    c. It is more common in the elderly.

    d. It is uninfluenced by corneal thickness.

22   What does increased intracranial pressure cause?

    a. optic neuritis
    b. ischemic optic neuropathy
    c. glaucoma
    d. papilledema

23.   What are 2 common ocular manifestations of myasthenia gravis?

    a. ptosis and diplopia
    b. proptosis and dry eye
    c. proptosis and uveitis
    d. ptosis and scleritis

24   What disease process is characterized by a reduction in blood flow to an organ or structure?

    a. neoplastic process
    b. metabolic process
    c. infectious process
    d. ischemic process

25   A patient with acquired immunity deficiency syndrome (AIDS) is least likely to have an eye infection caused by which of the following?

    a. histoplasmosis
    b. cytomegalovirus
    c. herpes zoster
    d. toxoplasmosis

26   A patient suffers from painful skin eruptions across the left side of his forehead that extends onto his left scalp area. What is the most likely condition?

    a. herpes simplex
    b. psoriasis
    c. varicella-zoster
    d. systemic histoplasmosis

27   What is the range of the wavelengths of visible light?

    a. 80 to 240 centimeters
    b. 400 to 750 nanometers
    c. 4 to 14 kilometers
    d. 360 to 490 millimeters

28   The surface of the normal eye is hydrophobic. What does this term mean?

    a. It is acidic.
    b. It is basic.

c. It resists water.

d. It is water friendly.

29 An exophthalmometer is used in screening for which of the following?

a. glaucoma

b. proptosis

c. strabismus

d. amblyopia

30 Which of the following patients would be best seen the same day that they call?

a. a patient previously diagnosed with cataract, with slowly progressive painless loss of vision in 1 eye over the prior 2 to 3 years

b. a patient with red and itchy eyes for the past month

c. a patient with sudden and total loss of vision in one eye ½ hour prior to calling

d. a patient with red eyes and drainage for the previous 2 to 3 days.

31 What is the material of choice for safety lenses?

a. chemically hardened glass

b. CR39 plastic

c. polycarbonate plastic

d. polyurethane plastic

32 Which statement is correct regarding visually impaired patients?

a. Verbal communication may be more extensive than with normally sighted patients.

b. Visually impaired patients will not benefit from a low-vision referral.

c. History-taking is the same as for normally sighted patients.

d. Visually impaired patients must be accompanied by a friend or family member.

33 Which of the following ophthalmic symptoms is most typical for a patient with new-onset diabetes mellitus?

a. flashing lights and floaters

b. intermittent droopy eyelids (ptosis)

c. blurred vision

d. dry eyes and dry mouth

34 Which of the following applies to a rigid protective eye shield?

a. protects a lacerated globe

b. prevents further bleeding

c. can be glued into place

d. prevents eyelid movement

35   A diabetic patient starts to have an acute hypoglycemic reaction in the office. What should the ophthalmic technician prepare to do besides notify the doctor?

    a. Check the pupils for symmetry.
    b. Give the patient a quick-acting sugary food.
    c. Call 911.
    d. Give the patient an antiemetic agent.

36   Which part of the eye is involved in focusing light?

    a. cornea
    b. aqueous humor
    c. vitreous
    d. retina

37   In which location do the optic nerve fibers cross?

    a. optic chiasm
    b. optic tracts
    c. lateral geniculate body
    d. visual cortex

38   If a patient asks you a question about a test result or diagnosis, what is the best action to take?

    a. Give the information to the patient.
    b. Refer the patient to the Internet.
    c. Refer the patient to the ophthalmologist.
    d. Tell the patient you don't know the answer to the question.

39   All **except** which of the following are important in assessing a patient with glaucoma?

    a. measurement of intraocular pressure
    b. measurement of corneal thickness
    c. analysis of aqueous humor from the anterior chamber
    d. visual field examination

40   All **except** which of the following circumstances might require a pressure patch?

    a. a full-thickness corneal laceration
    b. a corneal abrasion
    c. a recently operated eye that has received a peribulbar anesthetic block
    d. a patient with an exposed eye from 7th cranial nerve palsy

41   Common causes of conjunctivitis include all **except** which of the following?

    a. bacteria
    b. allergy

    c. exposure to a sunlamp (UV light)

    d. viruses

42   Features of thyroid ophthalmopathy include all **except** which of the following?

    a. ptosis

    b. proptosis

    c. strabismus

    d. exposure keratopathy

43   The retina contains all **except** which of the following cells?

    a. goblet cells

    b. bipolar cells

    c. ganglion cells

    d. rod cells

44   The standard comprehensive eye examination includes all **except** which of the following?

    a. visual acuity

    b. intraocular pressure

    c. exophthalmometry

    d. slit-lamp examination

45   The uveal tract consists of all **except** which of the following?

    a. ciliary body

    b. inner limiting membrane

    c. choroid

    d. iris

46   What condition does **not** develop during adulthood?

    a. amblyopia

    b. macular degeneration

    c. cataract

    d. glaucoma

47   Which of the following is **not** a manifestation of rheumatoid arthritis?

    a. scleritis

    b. dry eye

    c. peripheral corneal ulceration

    d. follicular conjunctivitis

48   Which of the following is **not** correct regarding keratoconjunctivitis sicca?

    a. A dry mouth may be associated.
    b. Lubricants are often used for treatment.
    c. The lacrimal punctum should be dilated.
    d. The patient may have arthritis.

49   Which of the following is **not** found in the anterior segment of the eye?

    a. aqueous humor
    b. choroid
    c. Schlemm's canal
    d. lens

50   Which of the following is **not** part of the cardiovascular system?

    a. ophthalmic artery
    b. central retinal vein
    c. aqueous vein
    d. carotid artery

51   Which of the following is **not** part of the ophthalmic medical assistant's responsibilities?

    a. Estimate visual acuity.
    b. Measure intraocular pressure.
    c. Diagnose a condition.
    d. Take a history.

52   Which of the following is **not** part of the triage process?

    a. determining the nature of the patient's complaint
    b. determining the severity of the patient's complaint
    c. determining the duration of the patient's complaint
    d. a medical review of systems

53   Which of the following steps does **not** apply to the process of applying a pressure patch to the eye?

    a. The eye is anesthetized.
    b. A folded patch is used.
    c. Tape is placed on the forehead.
    d. The cheek is pulled up toward the forehead.

54   Which of the following structures is **not** found in the normal eyelid?

    a. bulbar conjunctiva
    b. orbicularis oculi muscle
    c. cilia
    d. meibomian glands

55   Which of the following structures is **not** involved in creating a focused visual image?

    a. lens
    b. cornea
    c. vitreous
    d. retina

56   Which of the following structures is **not** involved in the drainage of tears?

    a. canaliculus
    b. punctum
    c. nasolacrimal duct
    d. accessory lacrimal gland

57   Which of the following substances is **not** a hormone produced by the endocrine system?

    a. insulin
    b. cholesterol
    c. estrogen
    d. thyroxine

58   Which statement is **incorrect** concerning herpes simplex virus?

    a. It causes a corneal infection characterized by a dendritic pattern.
    b. It causes fever blisters or "cold sores."
    c. Corneal infection can lead to scarring.
    d. It causes shingles.

59   Which statement is **incorrect** regarding diabetes mellitus?

    a. Diabetes can affect peripheral nerves, kidneys, and eyes.
    b. Diabetes is a common cause of blindness.
    c. Diabetic retinopathy risk is not altered by a higher blood pressure and hemoglobin A_{1C} level.
    d. Laser treatment is an effective treatment for diabetic retinopathy.

60   Which statement is **incorrect** regarding HIV infection and AIDS?

    a. Human immunodeficiency virus (HIV) can be transmitted only by sexual contact.
    b. Cytomegalovirus (CMV) retinitis is a common ocular manifestation of acquired immunodeficiency syndrome (AIDS).
    c. Antiretroviral drugs prolong the life of AIDS patients.
    d. AIDS-related infections occur most commonly in patients with CD4 lymphocyte counts less than 50.

61   Which of the following is **not** an ocular manifestation of a systemic disease?

    a. glaucoma
    b. diabetic retinopathy
    c. Sjögren syndrome
    d. proptosis with exposure keratopathy

12 | OPHTHALMIC IMAGING

1   Which of the following images depicts the fundus camera?

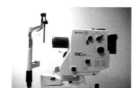
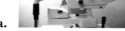
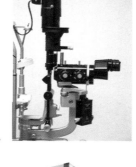

a.   **b.**

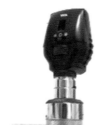
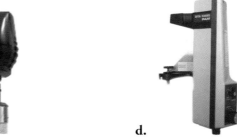

c.   **d.**

2   The most accurate method of performing a B-scan ultrasound is through what approach?

    a. with the probe and ultrasound gel in direct contact on the closed eyelid
    b. with the probe held over the area of interest, but not in direct contact with the patient
    c. with the probe and ultrasound gel in direct contact on the surface of the anesthetized eye
    d. with the probe without ultrasound gel in direct contact on the surface of the anesthetized eye

3   What is the best photographic test to document the size, appearance, and location of an atypical choroidal nevus?

    a. fundus photography
    b. external photography

    c. slit-lamp photography
    d. specular microscopy photography

4   What is the function of angling the slit beam in slit-lamp photography?

    a. serves as the gold-standard for measuring corneal thickness
    b. allows one to see deeper into the eye
    c. provides visualization of the limbus
    d. provides an appreciation of depth

5   What is the function of the corneal endothelial cells?

    a. prevents the entrance of bacteria, viruses, and fungi into the eye
    b. acts as a pump to keep fluid out of the corneal layers to keep it clear
    c. maintains elasticity of the cornea to protect it from damage
    d. produces fluid to the keep the anterior chamber formed

6   What test uses concentric lighted rings (Placido disks) to visually and quantitatively depict the amount of astigmatism present in the cornea?

    a. corneal topography
    b. specular microscopy
    c. slit-lamp photography
    d. scanning laser polarimetry (GDx)

7   What type of photography requires a close-up lens with an electronic flash attachment?

    a. fundus photography
    b. external photography
    c. corneal topography
    d. scanning laser polarimetry

8   A fundus fluorescein angiogram typically highlights details of the retinal vasculature. Fundus indocyanine green (ICG) angiography typically highlights details of what vascular system?

    a. iris vasculature
    b. choroidal vasculature
    c. optic nerve vasculature
    d. ciliary body vasculature

9   Patients undergoing intravenous fundus fluorescein angiography frequently report what common side effect?

    a. dizziness
    b. chest pain
    c. tingling in their hands and feet
    d. nausea

10   Intravenous fundus fluorescein angiography is the test that is most helpful in determining the presence or absence of which of the following?

a. guttata
b. retinal or choroidal neovascularization
c. meibomian gland dysfunction
d. phlyctenules

11   Pharmacologic dilation of the pupil (mydriasis) is absolutely required for which of the following tests?

a. fundus photography
b. optical coherence tomography
c. external photography
d. slit-lamp photography

12   Slit-lamp photography is useful for documentation of which of the following?

a. structure of the anterior chamber of the eye
b. optic nerve notch
c. ciliary body cysts
d. retinal blood vessel abnormalities

13   The Heidelberg retinal tomograph (HRT), optical coherence tomography (OCT), and GDx scanning laser polarimeter with variable corneal compensation are all used to measure what finding and assess what condition?

a. retinal thickness; pseudophakic cystoid macular edema
b. retinal thickness; age-related macular degeneration
c. retinal nerve fiber layer thickness; diabetic retinopathy
d. retinal nerve fiber layer thickness; glaucoma

14   What individuals need to be present to perform intravenous fundus fluorescein or indocyanine green (ICG) angiography?

a. registered nurse only
b. ophthalmic assistant and photographer
c. physician with or without a photographer
d. photographer only

15   What tests are the most helpful in confirming the diagnosis of a full-thickness macular hole?

a. optical coherence tomography and fundus photography
b. optical coherence tomography and B-scan (B-mode) ultrasonography
c. optical coherence tomography and intravenous fundus fluorescein angiography
d. optical coherence tomography and intravenous indocyanine green angiography

16   Which of the following is fluorescein angiography most helpful at characterizing?

     a. drusen
     b. retinal detachment
     c. myelinated nerve fiber
     d. vascular obstruction of blood vessels

17   Which of the following relationships is correct?

     a. A-scan ultrasonography and lensometry
     b. A-scan ultrasonography and biometry
     c. specular microscopy and keratometry
     d. specular microscopy and pachymetry

18   Which ophthalmic imaging test employs light to create a cross-sectional image of the retina using false coloration?

     a. A-scan (A-mode) biometry
     b. B-scan (B-mode) echography
     c. optical coherence tomography (OCT)
     d. intravenous fundus fluorescein angiography

19   Indocyanine green angiography is used specifically to study what part of the eye?

     a. angle structure of the eye
     b. zonular structure of the eye
     c. iris structure of the eye
     d. choroidal circulation of the eye

20   Which of the following tests should **not** be used if a patient has a documented history of shellfish or iodine allergies?

     a. fluorescein angiography
     b. indocyanine green angiography
     c. slit-lamp photography
     d. applanation tonometry

21   Which of the following is **not** a common side effect of fluorescein angiography?

     a. severe allergic reaction
     b. hives
     c. nausea
     d. yellow coloration of the urine

22   What types of images are **not** obtained with a fundus camera with angiography capabilities?

     a. 35-mm film color fundus photographs
     b. digital color fundus photographs

    c. 35-mm film color fundus fluorescein angiography images
    d. digital black-and-white fluorescein angiography images

13 | REFRACTOMETRY

1   Patients with hyperopia may see more clearly with what kind of lens?

    a. plus power diverging lens
    b. minus power diverging lens
    c. plus power converging lens
    d. minus power converging lens

2   In a myopic eye, where are images of distant objects focused?

    a. on the retina
    b. in front of the retina
    c. behind the retina
    d. 1 mm posterior to the crystalline lens

3   Why is retinoscopy used?

    a. to check for vitreous floaters
    b. to inspect the retina
    c. to find the fixation point of the eye
    d. to objectively estimate the refractive error of the eye

4   A cylindrical lens corrects what type of refractive error?

    a. myopia
    b. hyperopia
    c. astigmatism
    d. presbyopia

5   What is the focal length of a 3.00 D convex lens?

    a. 0.33 m
    b. 0.1 m
    c. 1.0 m
    d. 3.0 m

6   Where is the focal point of a hyperopic eye located?

    a. in front of the retina
    b. on the retina
    c. behind the retina
    d. in front of the lens

7   The axis of a cylinder is located how many degrees from its meridian of curvature (power)?

    a. 30°
    b. 60°
    c. 90°
    d. 180°

8   A toric lens is the same as which of the following?

    a. sphere
    b. vertex
    c. spherocylinder
    d. prism

9   What geometric term refers to the clearest image between the 2 focal points of a spherocylinder lens?

    a. refractive index
    b. circle of least confusion
    c. principal meridian
    d. add

10   The focal point of light rays in the figure represents an eye with what refractive error?

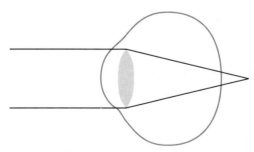

(Reproduced, with permission, from Newmark E, *Ophthalmic Medical Assisting: An Independent Study Course,* 4th ed, American Academy of Ophthalmology, 2006.)

    a. myopia
    b. hyperopia
    c. presbyopia
    d. emmetropia

11   What is the diopter power of a convex lens with a focal length of 40 centimeters?

    a. +5.00 D
    b. +1.00 D
    c. +0.20 D
    d. +2.50 D

12   All of the following **except** which step are part of refractometry?

    a. refinement
    b. binocular balance
    c. transposition
    d. retinoscopy

13   Regarding a cross cylinder lens, all phrases below are correct **except** which of the following?

    a. consists of cylinders of equal power, a minus and a plus lens with their axis at 90° from each other
    b. used to refine the correct axis of the cylindrical lenses to treat astigmatism
    c. used to refine the correct power of the cylindrical lenses to treat astigmatism
    d. used to refine the correct power of the near vision lenses to treat presbyopia

14   Refractometry includes all of the following **except** which step?

    a. binocular balancing
    b. lensometry
    c. retinoscopy
    d. refinement

14 | SPECTACLE SKILLS

1   Eyeglasses with what type of lens may correct diplopia (double vision)?

    a. prism lens
    b. spherocylinder in each lens
    c. plus lens in the dominant eye and a minus lens in the nondominant eye
    d. lenses whose circle of least confusion falls on the retina in each eye

2   Which statement is correct regarding the following spectacle prescription? +2.25 +1.50 × 180 add +2.50

    a. The prescription is written for a trifocal.
    b. The prescription is for a patient with simple hyperopia.
    c. The transposed form would be +3.75 −1.50 × 90.
    d. The vertex distance needs to be included in this prescription.

3   How may transposition of an eyeglass prescription be used?

    a. to move the optical centers of the lenses away from the pupils
    b. to change the position of the bifocal in a lens
    c. to convert a minus cylinder power to a plus cylinder power
    d. to specify the distance from the eye to the back surface of the eyeglass lens

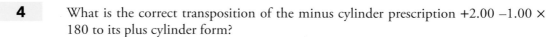

4   What is the correct transposition of the minus cylinder prescription +2.00 −1.00 × 180 to its plus cylinder form?

    a. +1.00 +1.00 × 180
    b. +3.00 +1.00 × 90
    c. +1.00 +1.00 × 90
    d. +2.00 +1.00 × 90

5   Which statement is correct regarding eyeglass frame adjustment?

    a. Optical centers should be in front of the center of the pupils.
    b. Pantoscopic tilt should be avoided.
    c. Segment height is important only for lined bi- and trifocals.
    d. Optical centers may be corrected by pantoscopic tilt.

6   Which statement is correct regarding the base curve of an eyeglass lens?

    a. A Geneva lens clock measures only base curve of a glass lens (not plastic).
    b. The base curve is determined by the lens power.
    c. Changing base curve will not be uncomfortable if it is symmetric.
    d. The base curve is measured on the front surface of the lens.

7   Which statement is correct regarding multifocal spectacle lenses?

    a. Modern progressive-addition lenses have a high patient satisfaction rate.
    b. Invisible or blended bifocals provide good intermediate-distance vision.
    c. Round top segments are increasingly popular.
    d. Patients may not change from lined to progressive-addition multifocal lenses.

8   Which statement is correct regarding eyeglass lenses?

    a. Photochromic lenses must be made of glass.
    b. Lenses may be cleaned without damage by using proper methods and materials.
    c. Polarized lenses do not protect the wearer from UVA or UVB rays.
    d. Antireflective coatings improve appearance but not vision.

9   What type of eyeglass lenses reduce glare?

    a. tinted lenses
    b. antireflective-coated lenses
    c. photochromic lenses
    d. polarized lenses

10   In most eyeglasses, the monocular pupillary distance for near vision will be less than the monocular pupillary distance for far vision by what amount?

    a. less than 1 millimeter
    b. about 2 millimeters

c. about 4 millimeters
d. about 6 millimeters

11   What is used to measure the vertex distance of a pair of eyeglasses?

a. small millimeter ruler
b. Geneva lens gauge
c. caliper
d. vertex distance comparison card

12   Which statement is correct regarding measurements used to fit eyeglasses?

a. The base curve is the back curve of the lens surface.
b. The near pupillary distance is required to manufacture all eyeglasses.
c. The vertex distance is the distance from the back surface of the lens to the cornea.
d. The optical center varies depending on vertex distance.

13   What does a Geneva lens clock measure?

a. pantoscopic angle
b. base curve
c. segment height
d. optical center

14   What is the recommended height of a bifocal segment?

a. dissecting the pupil
b. lower lid margin
c. 5 mm below the lower lid
d. 5 mm above the lower lid margin

15 SUPPLEMENTAL SKILLS

1   In measuring axial length, what is the most common cause of error?

a. a short axial length due to compression of the cornea with contact A-scan ultrasonography
b. a poor echo due to a dry cornea when measuring with contact A-scan ultrasonography
c. a short axial length due to compression of the sclera by the immersion scan shell
d. a long axial length due to an off-axis scan with immersion A-scan ultrasonography

2   What is the test called that places a strip of filter paper in the outer lower fornix of the eye?

    a. gonioscopy
    b. corneal sensitivity
    c. Schirmer
    d. Worth 4-dot

3   What is the minimal tear-film breakup time considered normal?

    a. 3 seconds
    b. 6 seconds
    c. 10 seconds
    d. 30 seconds

4   What is the average axial length of the human eye?

    a. 21.00 to 22.00 mm
    b. 23.00 to 23.50 mm
    c. 25.00 to 26.00 mm
    d. 26.00 to 28.00 mm

5   What is the normal thickness of the central cornea?

    a. 0.47 mm
    b. 0.56 mm
    c. 0.61 mm
    d. 0.68 mm

6   To estimate the anterior chamber depth, what is the first step?

    a. Shine a flashlight near the limbus from the temporal side of the eye.
    b. Shine a flashlight near the limbus from the nasal side of the eye.
    c. Shine a flashlight into the eye at an angle of 45°.
    d. Shine a flashlight directly into the eye.

7   Gonioscopy is used to examine which of the following?

    a. retina
    b. lens
    c. angle structure of the eye
    d. conjunctiva

8   What is a normal tear production measurement for a Schirmer test with topical anesthetic (Schirmer II)?

    a. more than 10 mm in 5 minutes
    b. more than 5 mm in 10 minutes
    c. more than 15 mm in 15 minutes
    d. more than 10 mm in 10 minutes

9   What does the phenol red thread test measure?

    a. color vision
    b. ocular pH
    c. corneal sensitivity
    d. tear output

10   Increased corneal thickness is commonly associated with which of the following?

    a. pingueculitis
    b. abnormalities of the corneal endothelial cells
    c. abnormalities of the corneal epithelial cells
    d. scleritis and episcleritis

11   How are ultrasonography units calibrated?

    a. by touching the probe to a test block specific for that machine
    b. by touching the probe to a flat surface
    c. by routinely measuring the same person's eye as a standard
    d. by pressing the instrument calibration button

12   A 65-year-old patient has the sensation of a foreign body in her eyes, as well as tearing and blurring of the eyes, especially in windy situations. What test would be most helpful for this patient?

    a. pinhole test
    b. indirect ophthalmoscopy
    c. Schirmer test
    d. visual field test

13   Most patients tested for glare sensitivity with the brightness acuity tester (BAT) have significant decrease in vision at what light intensity?

    a. low-medium
    b. medium
    c. medium-high
    d. high

14   What information is necessary to calculate the power of an intraocular lens?

    a. corneal thickness, axial length, and lens manufacturer's A constant
    b. corneal diameter, axial length, and lens manufacturer's A constant
    c. corneal curvature, patient's refractive error, lens manufacturer's A constant
    d. corneal curvature, axial length, and lens manufacturer's A constant

15   Which of the following will result from a 1-mm error in axial length measurement?

    a. approximately 3 D of change in postoperative refractive error
    b. approximately 2 D of change in postoperative refractive error

c. approximately 1 D of change in postoperative refractive error
d. no significant change in postoperative refractive error

16 Which device is used to measure corneal thickness?

a. tonometer
b. keratometer
c. phoropter
d. pachymeter

17 Which statement is **incorrect** regarding anterior chamber depth?

a. It is often shallower in a patient with nuclear sclerotic cataracts.
b. It is usually shallower in a patient with myopia than in a patient with hyperopia.
c. It may affect intraocular pressure.
d. It can be compressed when a contact A-scan probe is used.

16 | TONOMETRY

1 The examiner is preparing to measure intraocular pressure with the Goldmann applanation tonometer. Which of the following must be instilled into the eye, along with the topical anesthetic?

a. rose bengal
b. fluorescein
c. lissamine green
d. gentian violet

2 In the measurement of intraocular pressure (IOP) with the Goldmann applanation tonometer, the intraocular pressure is indicated by a number on the calibrated dial. This reading is multiplied by what number to express the IOP in millimeters of mercury?

a. 2
b. 5
c. 10
d. 20

3   A patient undergoing Goldmann tonometry has a central corneal thickness significantly thicker than average. What can be said of the endpoint shown in the figure?

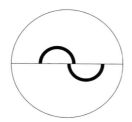

(Reproduced, with permission, from Newmark E, ed. *Ophthalmic Medical Assisting: An Independent Study Course,* 4th ed. San Francisco: American Academy of Ophthalmology; 2006.)

a. It is correct, but the reading is significantly higher than the actual intraocular pressure.
b. It is correct, but the reading is significantly lower than the actual intraocular pressure.
c. It is incorrect, and the examiner should adjust the knob so that the mires are spread apart.
d. It is incorrect, and the examiner should adjust the knob so that the mires are closer together.

4   What is a way the air-puff tonometer differs from the Goldmann tonometer?
a. It is an indentation tonometer.
b. It uses a red stain on the cornea.
c. It is a noncontact approach.
d. It always reads lower.

5   What is a disadvantage of the Goldman applanation tonometer?
a. It is not standardized.
b. It is not portable.
c. It is hard to sterilize.
d. Reproducibility of readings is poor.

6   What is a potential disadvantage of using the Schiøtz tonometer in a highly myopic eye?
a. The patient will squint because the instrument is in focus as it approaches the eye.
b. Myopic eyes are prone to corneal abrasions from the tip.
c. Intraocular pressure will be underestimated due to low scleral rigidity.
d. Intraocular pressure will be overestimated due to high scleral rigidity.

7   How should the plastic tip of an applanation tonometer be cleaned after use?
a. wiped with a clean tissue
b. soaked in 5% boric acid solution for 5 minutes, rinsed, and allowed to dry
c. soaked in a 1:10 solution of household bleach, rinsed, and allowed to dry
d. boiled for 3 minutes in sterile water

8   Which of the following variables can affect an applanation tonometry measurement?

    a. height of the patient
    b. gender of the patient
    c. corneal thickness
    d. anterior chamber depth

9   A patient is tending to squeeze the eye shut during applanation tonometry. Which of the following is most likely to result in satisfactory pressure readings?

    a. Explain to the patient the importance of keeping the eye open.
    b. Insert a speculum to keep the eye open.
    c. Hold both eyelids open with one hand.
    d. Use a cotton-tipped applicator to gently elevate the upper eyelid.

10   Which of the following has **no** effect upon the intraocular pressure reading obtained with the Goldmann applanation tonometer?

    a. corneal astigmatism
    b. corneal thickness
    c. external pressure on the eye from the examiner's fingers
    d. a tight collar or necktie

11   Which of the following tonometers does **not** provide a direct pressure reading in mm Hg?

    a. Schiøtz tonometer
    b. Goldmann tonometer
    c. Tono-Pen tonometer
    d. Air-puff tonometer

12   If the upper eyelid is resting on the applanation tonometer tip (unaware to the examiner), which of the following is **not** likely?

    a. The pressure will be underestimated.
    b. The pressure will be overestimated.
    c. An accurate reading will be obtained.
    d. The mires will be distorted.

13   Which of the following is **not** an applanation tonometer?

    a. Tono-Pen tonometer
    b. Perkins tonometer
    c. MacKay-Marg tonometer
    d. Schiøtz tonometer

17 VISUAL ASSESSMENT

1   What is the first procedure performed during the physical examination of a patient's eyes?

    a. discussion of the reason the patient has come to the ophthalmologist's office (chief complaint)
    b. measurement of visual acuity
    c. measurement of the intraocular pressure
    d. examination of the pupillary response

2   What does a pinhole acuity test confirm?

    a. The patient has a vitreous hemorrhage that is causing below-normal vision.
    b. The patient is legally blind.
    c. The patient is presbyopic.
    d. The patient has a refractive error that is the cause of below-normal vision.

3   Near vision is measured at what distance from the patient's eyes, unless specifically recorded otherwise?

    a. 6 inches
    b. 10 inches
    c. 14 inches
    d. 18 inches

4   Which of the following is a measure for visual acuity?

    a. the ability to see traffic clearly when driving a car
    b. the ability to read
    c. a Snellen chart
    d. the ability to follow a golf ball once hit

5   Visual acuity of 20/40 indicates that the patient sees which of the following?

    a. at 20 feet what a normal eye would see at 40 feet
    b. at 40 feet what a normal eye would see at 20 feet
    c. at 20 feet what a normal eye would see at 20 feet
    d. at 40 feet what a normal eye would see at 40 feet

6   Using the metric system, a vision of 6/24 is the same as which of the following?

    a. 20/24 in the English system
    b. 20/6 in the English system
    c. 20/60 in the English system
    d. 20/80 in the English system

7   What does the term *ocular media* refer to?

    a. the average vision considering both eyes
    b. the cornea and the retina
    c. a cataract
    d. the cornea, lens, and vitreous

8   Which phrase is accurate regarding cataract removal with intraocular lens implantation?

    a. is rarely performed
    b. can often restore vision to an excellent level
    c. is contraindicated with a dense white cataract
    d. is contraindicated to perform as an outpatient

9   Which of the following can affect the clarity of the cornea?

    a. scars and edema
    b. temporal arteritis
    c. cataract
    d. amblyopia

10   Which phrase accurately describes corneal transplantation?

    a. often restores excellent vision in patients with no light perception (NLP) vision
    b. often restores excellent vision in patients with corneal scars
    c. cannot restore vision in patient's with corneal edema
    d. should not be performed in the elderly

11   Which phrase is correct regarding visual potential tests?

    a. are an alternate method of measuring visual acuity
    b. grade the density of a cataract
    c. bypass opacities in the ocular media to measure the visual potential of the retina and optic nerve
    d. are inaccurate and should not be performed

12   What phrase applies to the potential acuity meter (PAM)?

    a. projects a Snellen acuity chart through a window in the media opacity
    b. must be performed with the pupil dilated
    c. works in cases of cataract but not for corneal scarring
    d. is rarely useful

13   Which phrase applies to contrast sensitivity testing?

    a. is unimportant
    b. is an important, but difficult part of the visual assessment

   c.   is important, and can be determined in an office setting
   d.   requires expensive and difficult-to-use equipment

14   Which phrase applies to the brightness acuity tester (BAT)?
   a.   is another way to test potential vision
   b.   is another way to measure best corrected visual acuity
   c.   is a method of demonstrating a patient's complaint regarding decreased visual
        acuity in bright light
   d.   determines whether a cataract operation will be successful

15   Which of the following statements applies to infants and young children?
   a.   They cannot have their vision assessed.
   b.   They should have their eyes tested quickly.
   c.   They require patience when being examined for visual assessment.
   d.   They should wait until they know the alphabet before seeing an
        ophthalmologist.

16   How should near acuity be measured?
   a.   without a lens in front of the eye and the near card held at 14 inches
   b.   with both eyes opened and reading a book in good lighting
   c.   monocularly with the distance correction with additional plus power lens
   d.   with a + 2.50 lens for each eye holding a near card at 14 inches

18 | VISUAL FIELDS

1   What is the term for an area of reduced sensitivity in the visual field?
   a.   isopter
   b.   scotoma
   c.   boundary
   d.   contour

2   The Amsler grid would be most helpful for a patient with which of the following?
   a.   cataract
   b.   glaucoma
   c.   retinal detachment
   d.   macular degeneration

3   The center of the island of vision corresponds to what part of the eye?

     a. lens
     b. iris
     c. pupil
     d. fovea

4   The visual information travels from the optic tracts to terminate in which part of the brain?

     a. frontal lobe
     b. temporal lobe
     c. parietal lobe
     d. occipital lobe

5   In what direction is the largest boundary of a normal visual field?

     a. temporally
     b. nasally
     c. superiorly
     d. inferiorly

6   What is the purpose of perimetry?

     a. to detect abnormalities in the visual field
     b. to detect cataractous changes
     c. to follow progression of a third cranial nerve palsy
     d. to diagnose congenital color defects

7   A patient undergoes computerized static perimetry. A certain area of the visual field in 1 eye fails to respond to the brightest stimulus available on the machine. What is this defect known as?

     a. absolute scotoma
     b. relative scotoma
     c. baring of the blind spot
     d. false positive response

8   Which of the following Goldmann stimuli would outline the largest isopter in a human eye?

     a. I_{4e}
     b. II_{4e}
     c. III_{4e}
     d. V_{4e}

9   What do the decibel numbers appearing on a visual field printout indicate?

     a. how loud the machine was during the stimulus presentations
     b. the actual location of the test points relative to fixation

c. how much the maximum available stimulus intensity had been dimmed to still elicit a response from the patient

d. how much the minimum available stimulus intensity had been turned up to elicit a response from the patient

10   What is the name of the visual field test that isolates the blue cone?

a. white-on-white perimetry
b. kinetic perimetry
c. short wavelength automated perimetry
d. frequency-doubling perimetry

11   A person with a bitemporal hemianopia is most likely to have what condition?

a. pituitary tumor
b. glaucoma
c. occipital brain tumor
d. cerebrovascular accident (stroke)

12   What is the most likely cause of a defect seen on a visual field that respects (does not cross) the vertical midline?

a. glaucoma
b. diabetic retinopathy
c. retinal scar
d. stroke

13   What kind of defect does damage to the macula typically produce?

a. arcuate scotoma
b. Bjerrum scotoma
c. nasal step
d. central scotoma

14   In the visual fields shown, the condition depicted is most likely due to what cause?

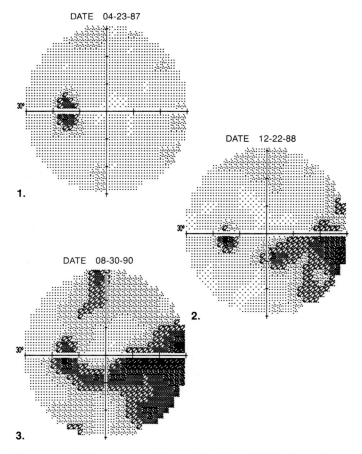

Progression of glaucomatous damage. The 3 visual fields shown illustrate the development and advancement of a visual field defect. Between the first and second visual fields, the patient developed a significant inferior nasal step. The third visual field illustrates the extension of this defect to the blind spot, as well as the development of a superior visual field loss (Humphrey 30–2 program). (Reproduced, with permission, from Cioffi GA, *Basic and Clinical Science Course*, Section 10: Glaucoma, American Academy of Ophthalmology, 2008–2009.)

a. macular degeneration
b. cataract
c. pituitary tumor
d. glaucoma

15   What does daily calibration of a perimeter ensure?

a. that patients will have similar test results each time
b. that room lighting is consistent
c. that the instrument has a consistent standard of sensitivity from day to day
d. that the perimeter's computer works each day

16   Which patient-related factors may improve the quality of a perimetry examination?

a. removing the chinrest
b. crying child in another room

c.   use of an automated perimeter

d.   presence of a perimetrist

17   What can be said of the all-white visual field result shown in the figure?

a.   It is acceptable, and the test does not need to be repeated.

b.   It indicates that the patient is not paying attention and not pushing the response button.

c.   It indicates that the patient does not understand the test and is constantly pushing the response button.

d.   It indicates possible glaucoma damage.

18   What factor affects the success of visual field testing?

a.   asking the patient to look at the fixation point

b.   asking the patient to follow the lights as they move

c.   moving the test object 4° per second

d.   keeping the room cold to help the patient stay awake

19   Two visual field tests from the same eye are performed sequentially on the same day. What is a possible explanation for the apparent improvement in the visual fields shown in the figure?

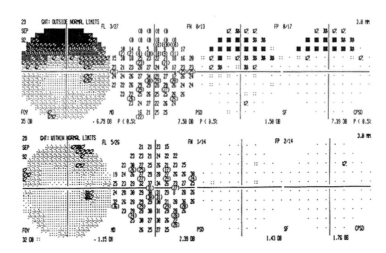

Two visual fields from the same eye performed sequentially on the same day. (Courtesy Neil T. Choplin, MD)

a.   The patient underwent a glaucoma procedure.

b.   The test was restarted after reinstructing the patient.

c.   The appropriate correcting lens was placed for the second test.

d.   The patient's upper eyelid was taped, correcting a ptosis.

20   Ptosis can affect what area of the visual field?

a.   superior

b. inferior

c. nasal

d. temporal

21 Two visual field tests from the same eye are performed sequentially on different days. In the figure, the result on the left was performed first. What is a possible explanation for the apparent improvement in the visual fields shown?

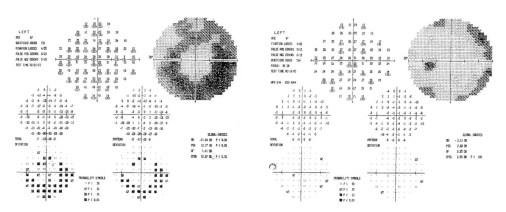

Two visual fields from the same eye performed sequentially on different days (the one on the left was performed first). (Courtesy Neil T. Choplin, MD)

a. The patient underwent a glaucoma procedure.

b. The patient was squinting during the first test.

c. The correcting lens was placed in the proper position for the second test.

d. The patient's upper eyelid was taped, correcting a ptosis.

22 Which of the following is **not** a specialized visual field test?

a. SWAP

b. Ishihara plates

c. frequency doubling technology

d. tangent screen

23 All **except** which of the following are methods for testing the visual field?

a. Amsler grid

b. confrontation

c. refractometry

d. computerized static perimetry

24 What is the most likely cause of a bitemporal visual field defect?

a. tumor near the chiasm

b. occipital lobe stroke

c. tumor near the optic radiations

d. aneurysm in the parietal lobe

19 | SURGICAL ASSISTING IN ASC OR HOSPITAL-BASED OR

1   Which laser is used to cut a hole in a cloudy posterior capsule after cataract surgery?

    a. excimer
    b. krypton
    c. carbon dioxide
    d. Nd:YAG

2   When should the surgical site be first identified?

    a. when the patient signs the consent form
    b. when the patient is brought to the operating room
    c. after the final surgical scrub is performed
    d. after a timeout is called just prior to the start of the surgery

3   Of the following, which suture material does the body break down?

    a. silk
    b. Mersilene
    c. polyglactin 910 (Vicryl)
    d. nylon

4   Of the sutures listed, which one is the largest diameter?

    a. 10–0
    b. 8–0
    c. 4–0
    d. 6–0

5   What medication is used prior to laser iridotomy?

    a. latanoprost
    b. glycerin
    c. timolol
    d. pilocarpine

6   Regarding nonrefractive laser therapy, which phrase is accurate?

    a. is performed only by retinal specialists
    b. cannot be used to treat glaucoma
    c. requires preparing a sterile field
    d. is noninvasive

7   Which laser is used to treat proliferative diabetic retinopathy?

    a. argon
    b. excimer
    c. Nd:YAG
    d. confocal

8   Laser safety includes all **except** which of the following guidelines?

    a. Always wear approved protective eye goggles when assisting the ophthalmologist.
    b. Never attempt to demonstrate how the laser works without the correct knowledge, permission, and supervision.
    c. Be sure to perform laser maintenance by yourself at appropriate dates.
    d. Review the instruction manual for specific safeguards before assisting in the laser work area.

9   Common types of ophthalmic lasers include all **except** which of the following?

    a. argon
    b. excimer
    c. Nd:YAG
    d. fluorescein

10   Steps to clean and protect surgical instruments after a procedure include all **except** which of the following?

    a. Remove all blood and tissues from disposable sharps before placing them in special sharps containers.
    b. Wear protective gloves.
    c. Cover delicate sharp instrument tips to reduce bends and misalignment and protect personnel.
    d. Count all sharps such as sutures, needles, and disposable blades to ensure none were left near the patient.

11   During a chalazion surgery, the ophthalmic medical assistant's duties may include all **except** which of the following?

    a. holding the clamp during the incision and curettage
    b. using a cellulose sponge to blot any blood
    c. passing a scalpel with the sharp end pointed toward the surgeon
    d. anticipating the surgeon's needs during the procedure

Certified Ophthalmic Assistant Exam Study Guide

Self-Assessment Answer Sheet

Record your responses to the questions in Section One on this answer sheet. Use the *Self-Assessment Answer Key* at the back of Section Two to score your work.

Category 1: History Taking

HIST 1 _____
HIST 2 _____
HIST 3 _____
HIST 4 _____
HIST 5 _____
HIST 6 _____
HIST 7 _____
HIST 8 _____

Category 2: Pupillary Assessment

PA 1 _____
PA 2 _____
PA 3 _____
PA 4 _____
PA 5 _____
PA 6 _____
PA 7 _____
PA 8 _____
PA 9 _____
PA 10 _____

Category 3: Equipment Maintenance and Repair

MAIN 1 _____
MAIN 2 _____
MAIN 3 _____
MAIN 4 _____
MAIN 5 _____
MAIN 6 _____
MAIN 7 _____
MAIN 8 _____
MAIN 9 _____
MAIN 10 _____
MAIN 11 _____
MAIN 12 _____
MAIN 13 _____
MAIN 14 _____
MAIN 15 _____
MAIN 16 _____
MAIN 17 _____
MAIN 18 _____
MAIN 19 _____
MAIN 20 _____

Category 4: Lensometry

LENS 1 _____
LENS 2 _____
LENS 3 _____
LENS 4 _____
LENS 5 _____
LENS 6 _____
LENS 7 _____
LENS 8 _____
LENS 9 _____
LENS 10 _____
LENS 11 _____
LENS 12 _____

Category 5: Keratometry

KERA 1 _____
KERA 2 _____
KERA 3 _____
KERA 4 _____
KERA 5 _____
KERA 6 _____
KERA 7 _____
KERA 8 _____
KERA 9 _____
KERA 10 _____

Category 6: Medical Ethics, Legal, and Regulatory Issues

ETHS 1 _____
ETHS 2 _____
ETHS 3 _____
ETHS 4 _____
ETHS 5 _____
ETHS 6 _____
ETHS 7 _____
ETHS 8 _____
ETHS 9 _____
ETHS 10 _____
ETHS 11 _____
ETHS 12 _____
ETHS 13 _____
ETHS 14 _____
ETHS 15 _____
ETHS 16 _____
ETHS 17 _____
ETHS 18 _____
ETHS 19 _____
ETHS 20 _____
ETHS 21 _____

Category 7: Microbiology

MICRO 1 _____
MICRO 2 _____
MICRO 3 _____
MICRO 4 _____
MICRO 5 _____
MICRO 6 _____

Category 8: Pharmacology

PHAR 1 _____
PHAR 2 _____
PHAR 3 _____
PHAR 4 _____
PHAR 5 _____
PHAR 6 _____
PHAR 7 _____
PHAR 8 _____
PHAR 9 _____
PHAR 10 _____
PHAR 11 _____
PHAR 12 _____
PHAR 13 _____
PHAR 14 _____
PHAR 15 _____
PHAR 16 _____
PHAR 17 _____
PHAR 18 _____
PHAR 19 _____
PHAR 20 _____
PHAR 21 _____
PHAR 22 _____
PHAR 23 _____
PHAR 24 _____
PHAR 25 _____
PHAR 26 _____
PHAR 27 _____
PHAR 28 _____
PHAR 29 _____
PHAR 30 _____
PHAR 31 _____
PHAR 32 _____

Category 9: Ocular Motility

MOTI 1 _____
MOTI 2 _____
MOTI 3 _____
MOTI 4 _____
MOTI 5 _____
MOTI 6 _____

Category 10: In-Office Minor Surgical Procedures

SURG 1 _____
SURG 2 _____
SURG 3 _____
SURG 4 _____
SURG 5 _____
SURG 6 _____
SURG 7 _____
SURG 8 _____
SURG 9 _____
SURG 10 _____
SURG 11 _____
SURG 12 _____
SURG 13 _____
SURG 14 _____
SURG 15 _____
SURG 16 _____

Category 11: Ophthalmic Patient Services and Education

PAT 1 _____
PAT 2 _____
PAT 3 _____
PAT 4 _____
PAT 5 _____
PAT 6 _____
PAT 7 _____
PAT 8 _____
PAT 9 _____
PAT 10 _____
PAT 11 _____
PAT 12 _____
PAT 13 _____
PAT 14 _____
PAT 15 _____
PAT 16 _____
PAT 17 _____
PAT 18 _____
PAT 19 _____
PAT 20 _____
PAT 21 _____
PAT 22 _____
PAT 23 _____
PAT 24 _____
PAT 25 _____
PAT 26 _____
PAT 27 _____
PAT 28 _____
PAT 29 _____
PAT 30 _____
PAT 31 _____
PAT 32 _____
PAT 33 _____
PAT 34 _____
PAT 35 _____
PAT 36 _____
PAT 37 _____
PAT 38 _____
PAT 39 _____
PAT 40 _____
PAT 41 _____
PAT 42 _____
PAT 43 _____
PAT 44 _____
PAT 45 _____
PAT 46 _____
PAT 47 _____
PAT 48 _____
PAT 49 _____
PAT 50 _____
PAT 51 _____
PAT 52 _____
PAT 53 _____
PAT 54 _____
PAT 55 _____
PAT 56 _____
PAT 57 _____
PAT 58 _____
PAT 59 _____
PAT 60 _____
PAT 61 _____

Category 12: Ophthalmic Imaging

IMAG 1 _____
IMAG 2 _____
IMAG 3 _____
IMAG 4 _____
IMAG 5 _____
IMAG 6 _____
IMAG 7 _____
IMAG 8 _____
IMAG 9 _____
IMAG 10 _____
IMAG 11 _____
IMAG 12 _____
IMAG 13 _____
IMAG 14 _____
IMAG 15 _____
IMAG 16 _____
IMAG 17 _____
IMAG 18 _____
IMAG 19 _____
IMAG 20 _____
IMAG 21 _____
IMAG 22 _____

Category 13: Refractometry

REF 1 _____
REF 2 _____
REF 3 _____
REF 4 _____
REF 5 _____
REF 6 _____
REF 7 _____
REF 8 _____
REF 9 _____
REF 10 _____
REF 11 _____
REF 12 _____
REF 13 _____
REF 14 _____

Category 14: Spectacle Skills

SPEC 1 _____
SPEC 2 _____
SPEC 3 _____
SPEC 4 _____
SPEC 5 _____
SPEC 6 _____
SPEC 7 _____
SPEC 8 _____
SPEC 9 _____
SPEC 10 _____
SPEC 11 _____
SPEC 12 _____
SPEC 13 _____
SPEC 14 _____

Category 15: Supplemental Skills

SUPP 1 _____
SUPP 2 _____
SUPP 3 _____
SUPP 4 _____
SUPP 5 _____
SUPP 6 _____
SUPP 7 _____
SUPP 8 _____
SUPP 9 _____
SUPP 10 _____
SUPP 11 _____
SUPP 12 _____
SUPP 13 _____
SUPP 14 _____
SUPP 15 _____
SUPP 16 _____
SUPP 17 _____

Category 16: Tonometry

TON 1 _____
TON 2 _____
TON 3 _____
TON 4 _____
TON 5 _____
TON 6 _____
TON 7 _____
TON 8 _____
TON 9 _____
TON 10 _____
TON 11 _____
TON 12 _____
TON 13 _____

Category 17: Visual Assessment

VA 1 _____
VA 2 _____
VA 3 _____
VA 4 _____
VA 5 _____
VA 6 _____
VA 7 _____
VA 8 _____
VA 9 _____
VA 10 _____
VA 11 _____
VA 12 _____
VA 13 _____
VA 14 _____
VA 15 _____
VA 16 _____

Category 18: Visual Fields

VF 1 _____
VF 2 _____
VF 3 _____
VF 4 _____
VF 5 _____
VF 6 _____
VF 7 _____
VF 8 _____
VF 9 _____
VF 10 _____
VF 11 _____
VF 12 _____
VF 13 _____
VF 14 _____
VF 15 _____
VF 16 _____
VF 17 _____
VF 18 _____
VF 19 _____
VF 20 _____
VF 21 _____
VF 22 _____
VF 23 _____
VF 24 _____

Category 19: Surgical Assisting in ASC or Hospital-Based OR

ASST 1 _____
ASST 2 _____
ASST 3 _____
ASST 4 _____
ASST 5 _____
ASST 6 _____
ASST 7 _____
ASST 8 _____
ASST 9 _____
ASST 10 _____
ASST 11 _____

Self-Assessment Answers and Explanations

1 HISTORY TAKING

1 Which of the following is part of a comprehensive medical history?

    a. past ocular history
    b. pachymetry
    c. biomicroscopy
    d. IOL calculation

ANSWER **a.** past ocular history

EXPLANATION The present illness, past history, social history, and family history are part of a comprehensive medical history. Pachymetry measures the corneal thickness and is not part of the history. Biomicroscopy is a slit-lamp exam and not part of the history. IOL calculation is a test performed to determine the power of the intraocular lens used in cataract surgery. (Newmark 2006, 114–116)

2 What is the definition of a chief complaint?

    a. the condition causing the visual problem
    b. the condition explaining the patient's complaint
    c. the reason causing the patient to seek care
    d. a serious medical problem from the patient's past medical history

ANSWER **c.** the reason causing the patient to seek care

EXPLANATION The chief complaint (in the patient's own words) is the patient's main reason for making the appointment. It can be a symptom or a recommended follow-up for a disease such as glaucoma or cataract. Determining the condition causing the patient's visual problem is goal of the exam. The condition explaining the patient's complaint is the end product of the exam (diagnosis). A serious medical problem from the patient's past history is important information to highlight but it is not the chief complaint. (Newmark 2006, 114, 281)

3   In what way should a patient's chief complaint be documented?

a. in the patient's own words
b. in the doctor's own words
c. in the technician's own words
d. in the patient's spouse's own words

ANSWER   a. in the patient's own words

EXPLANATION   The patient's chief complaint should be documented in the patient's own words. Questions asked of the patient should cover the main reason for the visit, the symptoms, when they began, and if they are getting worse. (Newmark 2006, 114, 117, 281)

4   If the patient comes to the exam room with a family member, how should the medical assistant proceed?

a. Take a history from the family member.
b. Ask the patient if the family member should be present for the visit.
c. Ignore the family member.
d. Ask the family member to leave the room.

ANSWER   b. Ask the patient if the family member should be present for the visit.

EXPLANATION   Family members can be an important source of information about a patient, but they can also intimidate a patient (or medical professional). Asking the patient if the family member should remain in the room is a good practice. (Newmark 2006, 117, 228)

5   If a small child is brought for a first exam by her mother (Mary Jones), what is the best way to address the patient's mother?

a. "Mom, what is the reason for today's visit?"
b. "Mary, what is the reason for today's visit?"
c. "Ms. Jones, what is the reason for today's visit?"
d. "Lady, what is the reason for today's visit?"

ANSWER   c. "Ms. Jones, what is the reason for today's visit?"

EXPLANATION   Although a medical practice may have a different standard and patients may have their own preferences, addressing this adult woman should be done politely, by last name. Ms. Jones may be married and prefer Mrs. Jones, but she will likely tell you if she prefers another title. Referring to her as "Mom," "lady," or "Mary" is less polite. (Newmark 2006, 117, 231)

6   Why is it important to specifically inquire about a patient's occupational and recreational activities?

    a. It may identify mutually enjoyable activities, such as hiking or golf.

    b. Patients may be engaging in activities that are dangerous without proper ocular protection.

    c. Patients enjoy providing personal details about their lives.

    d. These questions distract patients from long waits to see the doctor.

ANSWER   **b.** Patients may be engaging in activities that are dangerous without proper ocular protection.

EXPLANATION   Patients may not volunteer information about their recreational and occupational pursuits, and they may not realize those activities might pose a danger to their eyes or their health. Finding out that a patient is a part-time metalworker but never wears safety goggles is an important part of his health history. Knowing this information can give the ophthalmologist an opportunity to educate the patient about those health risks and to make recommendations for the patient to decrease those risks—in this case, by wearing safety goggles while working with metalworking tools. The other choices may actually be true, but they are clearly less important for the patient's health. (Newmark 2006, 115)

7   When a history of sexually transmitted disease or illegal drug use is obtained, what is the next recommended step?

    a. Write this information in the chart in red pen.

    b. Write this information on a separate piece of paper.

    c. Talk with co-workers about the patient's history.

    d. Omit this information from the patient's record entirely.

ANSWER   **b.** Write this information on a separate piece of paper.

EXPLANATION   Potentially sensitive information about a person's health raises troubling ethical issues. If the information may compromise the person's reputation, it warrants special care and it may be best for the interviewer to write it on a separate piece of paper for the ophthalmologist to review. If the doctor believes it to be important, he or she can add it to the patient's official record. Writing sensitive information in red pen may increase the chance of other people reading the information, so it should not be used. Talking with other people about the patient who have no need to know the information is unethical. Omitting the information entirely risks harm to the patient, because the information may be important for the patient's care. (Newmark 2006, 117)

8   While striking a metal bolt with a hammer, a patient developed severe pain after he felt something hit his eye. What type of injury would this most likely represent?

    a. chemical injury

    b. thermal injury

    c. penetrating injury

    d. toxin injury

ANSWER   **c.** penetrating injury

EXPLANATION   Trauma is a sudden injury to the eye or other parts of the body. The cause could be mechanical and result in a penetrating injury. Trauma could also be related to a toxin, such as an insect bite. Rapid damage to the eye can occur from a thermal injury, such as that caused by a burning ember, or a chemical injury, such as an acid splash into the eye. Safety eyeglasses can prevent or mitigate the damage in all of the situations listed here. (Newmark 2006, 114, 220)

2 PUPILLARY ASSESSMENT

1   Which of the following medications will have an effect on pupil size or reactivity?
- **a.** tropicamide eyedrops
- **b.** ciprofloxacin eyedrops
- **c.** artificial tears
- **d.** proparacaine eyedrops

ANSWER   **a.** tropicamide eyedrops

EXPLANATION   It is preferable to carefully check the responses of the pupil to light before putting any eyedrop medication in the eye. Pilocarpine, for instance, can decrease the size of the pupil, and both phenylephrine and tropicamide increase the pupillary size, making them useful prior to a dilated eye examination. If dilating drops are used before examining the pupils, the value of the exam is lost. Artificial tears, topical anesthetics (proparacaine), and antibiotics (ciprofloxacin) do not have an effect on pupil size or reactivity. (Newmark 2006, 83, 125)

2   Examining the pupillary reactions can help locate abnormalities in which of the following?
- **a.** lens
- **b.** optic nerve
- **c.** extraocular muscles
- **d.** conjunctiva

ANSWER   **b.** optic nerve

EXPLANATION   Abnormalities of pupillary reactions can point to problems in the iris muscle or nerve supply of the iris, optic nerve problems, severe retinal pathology, or problems affecting the brain and central nervous system. Lens problems, even very dense cataracts, do not typically affect pupillary reactions. Extraocular muscle problems and conjunctival diseases would not cause pupillary abnormalities. (Bradford 2004, 32, 143; Newmark 2006, 125)

3   When a light is shined into an eye, it is expected to cause the pupil on that side to constrict. Which reaction of the pupil does this test assess?

a. direct reaction
b. consensual reaction
c. delayed reaction
d. confrontational reaction

ANSWER   a. direct reaction

EXPLANATION   This describes a test of the direct response of the pupil. The consensual reaction is assessed by looking at the other eye's response to illumination in the first eye. The other choices do not describe reactions of the pupil. (Newmark 2006, 125–126)

4   The pupil of a patient's eye constricts when the other eye is illuminated but fails to constrict when it is illuminated directly. This is an example of which defect?

a. consensual reaction defect
b. paradoxical reaction defect
c. reverse pupillary defect
d. afferent pupillary defect

ANSWER   d. afferent pupillary defect

EXPLANATION   An afferent pupillary defect (APD) exists when the consensual pupillary reaction is present but the direct reaction is absent on the same side. Its presence indicates severe retinal pathology or optic nerve disease. Consensual, paradoxical, and reverse defects do not describe the APD pupil. (Bradford 2004, 32, 143; Newmark 2006, 125)

5   Once pupils are dilated for a retinal exam, what can be stated about the pupillary reactions?

a. They are no longer reliable.
b. They should be easier to test.
c. They indicate intracranial pathology.
d. They may suggest drug abuse.

ANSWER   a. They are no longer reliable.

EXPLANATION   Pupillary testing is always performed before instilling diagnostic dilating drops. Pharmacologically dilated pupils preclude further testing of pupil function until after the effects of the dilating agents have worn off. For tropicamide, the effect may persist for 3 to 12 hours; the dilating effect of atropine may persist for days. (Newmark 2006, 125, 134)

6   The size of the pupil may be measured easily using which method?

a. laser interferometer
b. magnetic resonance imaging (MRI)

c. computed tomography (CT)
d. ruler or gauge

ANSWER   d. ruler or gauge

EXPLANATION   A simple means of measuring pupil size is the ruler, which is often used in clinical practice to measure the diameter of the pupil. A pupil gauge is also commonly used, in which the examiner compares the size of a printed semicircle to the patient's pupil. MRI and CT are imaging technologies for various body parts, including the head and brain. The laser interferometer estimates visual potential in cases of media opacities. (Trobe 2006, 10)

7   An asymptomatic patient has been referred to the ophthalmologist for evaluation of anisocoria, or unequal pupil size. The examination confirms the finding that the right pupil is 1 mm larger than the left pupil, although both pupils show a normal direct response to light. What is the best next step to evaluate pupil function?

a. Test for consensual response of each pupil.
b. Use tropicamide drops to dilate each eye.
c. Use timolol maleate drops to constrict each pupil.
d. Test for paradoxical response of each pupil.

ANSWER   a. Test for consensual response of each pupil.

EXPLANATION   Testing for the direct and consensual pupil responses are important components of the examination. Normally, when light is shined in one eye, that eye constricts (direct reaction) and the other eye also constricts, even when light does not reach it (consensual reaction). After the direct response is checked, the consensual response should be checked next. Tropicamide dilates the pupil and prevents further pupillary assessment. Timolol maleate is used for intraocular pressure reduction, but its use is not related to the pupil exam. Testing for "paradoxical reaction" to light is not part of the routine pupil examination. (Newmark 2006, 125)

8   A pupillary examination can evaluate which of the following?

a. nerve damage
b. glaucoma
c. cataract
d. scleral disease

ANSWER   a. nerve damage

EXPLANATION   Significant nerve damage will cause an afferent pupillary defect during a pupillary exam. Glaucoma causes an afferent pupillary defect late in the course of the disease only when significant nerve damage has occurred. Cataract and scleral disease do not cause pupillary abnormalities. (Newmark 2006, 125)

9   A light is shined into a patient's eye and the pupil of the other eye constricts. This is an example of which reaction?

    a. direct reaction
    b. paradoxical reaction
    c. confrontational reaction
    d. consensual reaction

ANSWER   **d.** consensual reaction

EXPLANATION   In the testing method for the consensual pupil response, an eye is illuminated and the response of the pupil in the other eye is assessed. Direct reaction is caused by light shined into the test eye. The confrontational reaction does not relate to a pupil reaction. Paradoxical reaction is an unexpected pupillary reaction. (Newmark 2006, 125)

10   During an examination of a new patient, an irregularly shaped pupil in one eye is noted. What is the best next course of action for the ophthalmic medical assistant?

    a. Dilate the patient's pupils.
    b. Discuss the findings with an ophthalmologist.
    c. Request anterior segment photographs.
    d. Perform cycloplegic retinoscopy.

ANSWER   **b.** Discuss the findings with an ophthalmologist.

EXPLANATION   The best practice is to check with the ophthalmologist about an abnormal pupil shape or size or reactivity, because it may be a sign of an ocular disease. Dilating the pupil is an incorrect response, because it would prevent the ophthalmologist from confirming the finding after the pupil has been dilated. While providing excellent documentation of the finding, photographing the pupil would not help with the patient's present management. Cycloplegic retinoscopy, which involves dilating the pupil, would prevent anyone else from seeing the pupillary abnormality until the drops wear off, hours later. This should not be performed until after the ophthalmologist has checked the pupils. (Newmark 2006, 125, 264)

3 EQUIPMENT MAINTENANCE AND REPAIR

1   Which of the following is a responsibility of ophthalmic medical assistants?

    a. Maintain the equipment directly used by themselves.
    b. Maintain the specific instruments they used that day.
    c. Clean only the instruments they use personally.
    d. Be responsible for all ophthalmic equipment whether they used the equipment themselves or not.

ANSWER   **d.** Be responsible for all ophthalmic equipment whether they used the equipment themselves or not.

EXPLANATION   Ophthalmic medical assistants are responsible for the care, maintenance, proper cleansing, and basic servicing of all ophthalmic equipment whether or not they personally had used them. (Newmark 2006, 285)

2   Which statement applies to optical lenses used in the ophthalmic practice?

   a. To prevent scratches they should not be cleaned.
   b. They can be cleaned with gauze soaked with saline solution.
   c. They can be cleaned with approved cleaning fluid.
   d. They can be cleaned with soft, dry facial tissue.

ANSWER   c. They can be cleaned with approved cleaning fluid.

EXPLANATION   Lenses must be free of oil, dust, dirt, and fingerprints in order to perform correctly. Always consult the lens manufacturer's manual and office policies regarding the cleaning of optical lenses. Never rub a dry lens. To prevent scratches, only use approved cleaning fluids and special lens cleaning papers or cloths. (Newmark 2006, 286)

3   Which statement applies to the Hruby lens?

   a. It allows a binocular view of the central fundus.
   b. It allows magnification of the peripheral fundus.
   c. It can be left in the same position after use.
   d. It should be soaked in solution in between each use.

ANSWER   a. It allows a binocular view of the central fundus.

EXPLANATION   The Hruby lens is a minus 55 D lens attached to the slit lamp (figure). It allows a binocular and magnified view of the vitreous and central fundus, and it is not used for the peripheral fundus exam. To avoid damage, after use the lens should be returned to its storage position on the slit lamp. The lens needs no soaking after use, as it does not contact the eye. (Newmark 2006, 286)

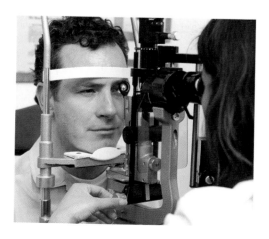

Hruby lens in use. (Reproduced, with permission, from Wilson FM, ed. *Practical Ophthalmology*, 6th ed. San Francisco: American Academy of Ophthalmology; 2009.)

4   What range of hand-held, noncontact, funduscopic lenses is used in conjunction with the slit lamp?

    a. +20 D to +40 D
    b. +60 D to +90 D
    c. +40 D to +60 D
    d. +20 D to +50 D

ANSWER   **b.** +60 D to +90 D

EXPLANATION   Hand-held, noncontact, funduscopic lenses used in conjunction with the slit lamp include +60, +78, +90. The lenses between +14 and +40 are used for indirect ophthalmoscopy. (Newmark 2006, 286)

5   If an electrical instrument fails to work, which of the following should be initiated first?

    a. Confirm that the instrument is plugged into the electric wall outlet.
    b. Call a licensed electrician.
    c. Change the fuse.
    d. Call the doctor to the room.

ANSWER   **a.** Confirm that the instrument is plugged into the electric wall outlet.

EXPLANATION   Troubleshooting an electric instrument failure is a common occurrence. The following checklist is helpful to correct the problem: (1) check the wall outlet plug; (2) check all connecters to the instrument; (3) check the bulb; (4) check the instrument fuse; and (5) check for a central circuit failure. (Newmark 2006, 289)

6   The phoropter is associated with which of the following features?

    a. It is used to perform a subjective lensometry.
    b. It is available only with nondisposable shields that need to be cleaned between uses.
    c. It should be cleaned front and back with alcohol and a soft, dry cloth.
    d. It should be scheduled for maintenance every 2 years.

ANSWER   **d.** It should be scheduled for maintenance every 2 years.

EXPLANATION   The phoropter is used to perform a manual subjective refraction. It comes in different varieties and brands, some with shields that need to be cleaned or some with disposable shields that are discarded between uses. The lenses should be cleaned front and back with lens paper or air, depending if the lens is exposed or enclosed. Alcohol should never be used on any part of the phoropter. Scheduled maintenance is every 2 years. Lensometry is the measurement of the power of the sphere and cylinder of an optical lens and the axis of the cylinder. The lensmeter is used for this determination. (Newmark 2006, 290)

7   If the slit-lamp light does not operate, what should the technician do?

    a. Check the electrical wall outlet plug and the instrument fuse and bulb.
    b. Check the internal transformer connections.
    c. Do not replace the bulb if it seems to be in good condition.
    d. Call the doctor to the room.

ANSWER   **a.** Check the electrical wall outlet plug and the instrument fuse and bulb.

EXPLANATION   Troubleshooting for a nonoperative slit lamp consists of checking the wall electric outlet plug, instrument fuse, and bulb. Check all external connections to the transformer. Do not open the transformer to examine the internal connections. After checking the electric connections and the lamp is still not working, replace the bulb even if it seems to be in good condition, using the manufacturer's guidelines. Lastly be certain the central electric circuit is functioning. (Newmark 2006, 292; Ledford 2006, 18)

8   Which of the following instruments provides a stereoscopic view of the retina?

    a. direct ophthalmoscope
    b. retinoscope
    c. gonioscope
    d. head-mounted indirect ophthalmoscope

ANSWER   **d.** head-mounted indirect ophthalmoscope

EXPLANATION   A binocular indirect ophthalmoscope (figure) is a head-mounted instrument that shines a light through a handheld lens into the patient's eye. The lens system allows an inverted image of the retina viewed stereoscopically. A direct ophthalmoscope requires that the examiner look through it with 1 eye, which does not allow a stereoscopic view. A retinoscope is an instrument for objective refractometry and is not used to view the retina. A gonioscope used with the slit lamp allows a stereoscopic view of the anterior chamber angle. (Newmark 2006, 135)

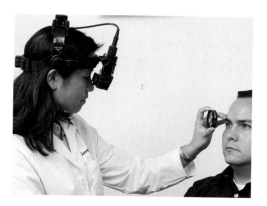

Ophthalmoscopic examination with the indirect ophthalmoscope. (Reproduced, with permission, from Wilson FM, ed. *Practical Ophthalmology,* 6th ed. San Francisco: American Academy of Ophthalmology; 2009.)

9   Care of the Snellen chart projector unit includes which of the following steps?

    a. Clean the slides with warm water or cleansing solutions.
    b. Clean the viewing mirrors with lint-free cloth or compressed air.

    c. Wait until the bulb goes completely dark before replacing it.

    d. Clean the external lens surfaces and focusing tubes once every 2 years to ensure they are clear.

ANSWER   **b.** Clean the viewing mirrors with lint-free cloth or compressed air.

EXPLANATION   The external lens surfaces and tubes should be cleaned at appropriate intervals to prevent dust accumulation, much more often than every 2 years. The glass slides should never be cleaned with water or other agents; only with dry photographic lens paper. The bulbs should be replaced when they start going dim to help ensure accurate testing. (Newmark 2006, 292–293)

10   Which of the following statements applies to the tip of the Goldmann-type tonometer?

    a. The prism tip contacts the eye and flattens a small area of the sclera by a known pressure or force.

    b. The prism tip should be thoroughly cleaned with an alcohol sponge and allowed to air dry.

    c. The prism tip should be cleansed by soaking with 10% hydrogen peroxide or regular household bleach.

    d. The prism tip can be used immediately after soaking.

ANSWER   **b.** The prism tip should be thoroughly cleaned with an alcohol sponge and allowed to air dry.

EXPLANATION   The Goldmann-type tonometer measures the intraocular pressure by flattening a small area of the cornea by a known pressure or force. The tip should be thoroughly cleaned with an alcohol sponge or cleansed with a 3% hydrogen peroxide soak for 5 minutes. Also, a 1:10 household bleach solution diluted with water may be used for 5 minutes. The tip should never be used immediately after soaking or wiping. It must first be rinsed and allowed to dry before coming in contact with a patient's cornea. (Newmark 2006, 294)

11   What is the proper way to care for a Tono-Pen?

    a. Clean the metal tip periodically of debris with compressed air.

    b. Clean the latex cover between each use.

    c. Store the unit without the tip covered.

    d. Replace the batteries whenever the readout displays "BAD."

ANSWER   **a.** Clean the metal tip periodically of debris with compressed air.

EXPLANATION   The metal tip should be cleaned periodically with compressed air. The latex sanitary cover is disposable and must always be discarded after each patient use. The instrument should be stored with the metal tip covered with a protective cap. Before replacing the batteries, try the RESET button first. (Newmark 2006, 295)

12   Common types of ophthalmic lasers include which of the following?

    a. argyle
    b. kryptonian
    c. exciser
    d. neodymium:yttrium-aluminum garnet

ANSWER   **d.** neodymium:yttrium-aluminum garnet

EXPLANATION   Common laser types used in the practice of ophthalmology are argon, krypton, excimer, diode, and Nd:YAG lasers (neodymium:yttrium-aluminum garnet), commonly called the *YAG*. (Newmark 2006, 296)

13   The manual lensmeter unit includes an eyepiece, lens holder, light source, and adjustment knobs. Proper maintenance of the unit includes which step?

    a. Blow dust from the lens surfaces with a clean, dry bulb syringe or compressed air.
    b. Wipe the external enamel finish with a jeweler's polishing cloth to prevent buildup.
    c. Lubricate the instrument if it feels tight.
    d. Use lens cleanser or detergent to clean the lens surfaces.

ANSWER   **a.** Blow dust from the lens surfaces with a clean, dry bulb syringe or compressed air.

EXPLANATION   Proper maintenance of the manual lensmeter includes blowing dust from the lens surfaces, wiping the external enamel finish with a soft cloth for dust collection, and calling a service technician if the instrument feels tight. Do not lubricate the instrument yourself. (Newmark 2006, 290–291)

14   Which statement is **incorrect** about the medical assistant's participation in the care of ophthalmic lenses and equipment?

    a. The medical assistant should calibrate the automated computerized perimeter on a daily basis.
    b. Basic care is the responsibility of the medical assistant.
    c. Items should remain clean and in good working condition in order to function reliably.
    d. The medical assistant should calibrate the laser instruments once yearly.

ANSWER   **d.** The medical assistant should calibrate the laser instruments once yearly.

EXPLANATION   The ophthalmic medical assistant often has the responsibility of caring for, maintaining, and performing basic servicing of ophthalmic equipment in the office. Many of the lenses and instruments used in an ophthalmology practice are delicate and costly. In addition, these items should remain clean and in good working condition to reliably perform their diagnostic or other medical function. Laser instruments should never be serviced or calibrated by a medical assistant. The automatic and manual perimeters should be calibrated once before use for the day. (Newmark 2006, 285–297)

15   Guidelines for cleaning noncontact lenses and mirrored surfaces include all **except** which of the following?

    a. Remove debris from lenses with an approved liquid by rubbing them with a lint-free cleaning cloth.

    b. Rub the lenses in a circular fashion to remove oils and fingerprints.

    c. Clean the lens at the first signs of dirt or debris.

    d. Thoroughly clean the optical mirrors with a dry lint-free cloth.

ANSWER   **d.** Thoroughly clean the optical mirrors with a dry lint-free cloth.

EXPLANATION   Thorough cleaning of optical mirrors in ophthalmic instruments, including the disassembly of any complex lens system, is a job for the instrument specialist or manufacturer's technician. For routine cleaning, the assistant can use a puff of air from a compressed-air can or a clean bulb syringe. A dry lens should never be rubbed clean. When using a recommended liquid cleaning agent, the assistant should gently rub the lens in a circular motion. No residue should be left to cloud the lens after cleaning. Lenses should be cleaned on a routine basis, not waiting for someone to become aware of the problem. (Newmark 2006, 286–287)

16   Guidelines for care of electrically powered instruments include all **except** which of the following?

    a. Cover instruments with a dust cover when not in use.

    b. Turn off everything in the exam rooms when not in use, except instruments being re-charged.

    c. Unplug equipment when performing any servicing except changing bulbs.

    d. Handle all bulbs with lens tissue paper to prevent oils from etching the bulb once it heats up.

ANSWER   **c.** Unplug equipment when performing any servicing except changing bulbs.

EXPLANATION   Guidelines for the care of electrically powered instruments include covering equipment and handling bulbs properly to prevent oils from building up and diminishing the bulbs' effectiveness. Instruments should be turned off when they are not in use to prolong the life of bulbs and batteries, except hand-held battery re-chargers. For safety, equipment should always be disconnected from the power source when being serviced, and even when changing the bulbs. (Newmark 2006, 289)

17   Which of the following lenses **does not** contact the eye?

    a. goniolens

    b. Koeppe lens

    c. 3-mirror fundus lens

    d. Hruby lens

ANSWER   **d.** Hruby lens

EXPLANATION   Lenses that contact the eye and need proper cleansing are the goniolens, the Koeppe lens, and a 3-mirror fundus lens. The Hruby lens is attached to the slit lamp and does not contact the eye. (Newmark 2006, 286–287)

18   What guideline does **not** apply for cleaning lenses that make contact with the eye?

    a. Rinse them thoroughly with lukewarm water to remove contaminants.
    b. After cleaning, blot them dry with a paper towel.
    c. Disinfect or sterilize them between use.
    d. Sterilize lenses that are used during surgery or on a recently operated eye.

ANSWER   **b.** After cleaning, blot them dry with a paper towel.

EXPLANATION   Lenses that make contact with the eye should be cleansed or sterilized based upon their use. Generally the lens should be cleaned immediately after contact with the eye, by rinsing the lens thoroughly with lukewarm water to remove contaminants. After cleaning or disinfection, the lenses can be blotted dry using a lint-free lens-cleaning paper or a soft lint-free absorbent lens cloth—not an ordinary paper towel, which can be abrasive enough to scratch the lens surface. Sterilization should follow standard procedures. (Newmark 2006, 287–288)

19   Which of the following is **not** considered a feature of the retinoscope?

    a. It is a hand-held instrument.
    b. It consists of a light source and a recording component.
    c. It is often powered by battery or rechargeable power packs.
    d. It is cleaned by blowing dust off the front surface with a clean bulb syringe.

ANSWER   **b.** It consists of a light source and a recording component.

EXPLANATION   The retinoscope is a hand-held, rechargeable instrument for objectively estimating a refractive error, consisting of a light source and a viewing component. It is used with either trial lenses or the phoropter to define a patient's refractive error before beginning subjective tests. It is cleaned by blowing dust off the front surface with compressed air or via a clean bulb syringe. (Newmark 2006, 289)

20   Regarding equipment maintenance and repair, which of the following is **not** performed by the ophthalmic medical assistant?

    a. cleaning lenses and equipment
    b. protecting instruments from dust and damage
    c. calibrating lasers
    d. replacing light bulbs and fuses

ANSWER   **c.** calibrating lasers

EXPLANATION   The ophthalmic assistant is often required to clean lenses and equipment, protect instruments from dust and damage, and replace light bulbs and fuses. Although the assistant may be asked to calibrate a tonometer, only qualified service technicians should perform maintenance on lasers. (Newmark 2006, 297)

4 LENSOMETRY

1
While checking progressive lens eyeglasses in a lensmeter, the technician notices that the lensmeter mires are centered on the third circle below the center of the lensmeter target by both lenses of the eyeglasses. What does this indicate?

a. The progressive lenses are in the lensmeter upside down.
b. There is base-down prism in both lenses of the eyeglasses.
c. The lensmeter is out of alignment.
d. The eyeglasses should be turned around to read the power from the other surface of the eyeglass lenses.

ANSWER   b. There is base-down prism in both lenses of the eyeglasses.

EXPLANATION   The circles in a manual lensmeter indicate prism power. If the intersection of the mires is below the center, the prism is base down. Similarly, the prism may be base up, base in, or base out if the intersection is decentered upward, toward the nose, or toward the temple. Equal base-down prism in each eye is often present in eyeglasses with progressive addition lenses. Distance power of the lenses is most accurately read with the back surface of the lens against the lensmeter. The power of the reading addition is most accurately read with the front surface of the lens against the lensmeter. (Newmark 2006, 73)

2
When looking through the eyepiece of a lensmeter, if the single line focuses at −4.00 D and the triple lines focus at −1.25D, what is the cylinder power?

a. −6.25 D
b. +2.75 D
c. +3.20 D
d. −2.75 D

ANSWER   b. +2.75 D

EXPLANATION   To determine the power of the cylinder, subtract the difference of the numerical value of 2 lens powers if they are both negative (eg, −4.00 D minus −1.25D equals 2.75 D). If 1 lens is negative and the other lens is positive, you would add the lens powers. (Newmark 2006, 71)

3
Which of the following is the correct order for a written eyeglass prescription?

a. sphere power, cylinder power, sphere axis
b. sphere power, cylinder axis, cylinder power
c. sphere power, cylinder power, cylinder axis
d. sphere power, sphere axis, cylinder power

ANSWER   c. sphere power, cylinder power, cylinder axis

EXPLANATION   The standard format used for writing an eyeglass prescription consists of the sphere power written first with the indicated prefix of plus (+) or minus (–) sign. If the prescription has no sphere power the word "plano" is used in the first notation. The sphere power or plano is followed next by the cylinder power with the accompanying prefix of plus or minus sign. The cylinder power is followed by the cylinder axis. A prescription without cylinder will contain only the sphere power. A prescription without sphere power but containing cylinder is written plano followed by the cylinder power and the axis. Typical examples follow. (Newmark 2006, 67–68)

$+1.50 +0.50 \times 090$ Plus sphere with plus cylinder and axis
Plano -0.75×180 No sphere with minus cylinder and axis
$-3.00 +1.25 \times 075$ Minus sphere with plus cylinder and axis
$+2.25$ Plus sphere without cylinder
-5.00 Minus sphere without cylinder

4   Neutralizing optical lenses is accomplished by which process?
   a. refractometry
   b. lensometry
   c. retinoscopy
   d. pachymetry

ANSWER   b. lensometry

EXPLANATION   Refractometry is a subjective process using optical lenses to determine the refractive error of an eye. Retinoscopy determines the refractive error of an eye objectively using a retinoscope and optical lenses. Pachymetry measures the corneal thickness by utilizing a pachymeter. (Newmark 2006, 69)

5   What is the first step in determining the prescription of a pair of eyeglasses with the lensmeter?
   a. Clean the lenses before reading.
   b. Adjust the eyepiece of the instrument.
   c. Position the frame on the spectacle table with the temples away from you.
   d. Turn the power drum to focus the mires to zero.

ANSWER   b. Adjust the eyepiece of the instrument.

EXPLANATION   The first step in performing lensometry for all types of lenses is focusing the instrument eyepiece. Having a clean lens is nice but not essential. A soiled lens will not give you an erroneous reading but an unfocused eyepiece can lead to errors in measuring the power. After the eyepiece has been adjusted, the power drum is able to focus the mires at zero with a plano lens. Positioning the frame with the temples away from you is correct but it is not the first step to be taken when performing lensometry. (Newmark 2006, 69–71)

6   What statement about lensmeter measurement of prisms is true?

    a. It measures the power and orientation of the prism base.
    b. It measures only base up and base in prism.
    c. It measures only base down and base out prism.
    d. It measures the power and axis of the prism.

ANSWER   **a.** It measures the power and orientation of the prism base.

EXPLANATION   The lensmeter can determine the power and orientation of the prism base by utilizing the concentric circles within the lensmeter target. Base in, base out, base up, and base down are all revealed when present in an eyeglass lens. Axis relates to cylinder lenses and not prisms. (Newmark 2006, 73)

7   What statement is true about the optical center of a lens?

    a. The optical center of a lens is placed at the lower eyelid margin.
    b. The optical center of a lens is placed directly in front of the pupil.
    c. Lenses that are not optically centered can result in an off-axis prescription.
    d. The Geneva lens clock can determine the optical center of a lens.

ANSWER   **b.** The optical center of a lens is placed directly in front of the pupil.

EXPLANATION   The optical center of a lens is always placed directly in front of the patient's pupil. In a patient with normal eyelids the bifocal segment height and not the optical center is set at the lower eyelid margin. The lensmeter can accurately determine the optical center of a lens by positioning the mires in the center of the target and marking the center with the dotting device. The Geneva lens clock measures the base curve of a lens. A lens not correctly centered in front of the pupil will induce unwanted prism in the prescription. The axis is associated with cylinder lenses and is not altered by optical center decentration. (Newmark 2006, 73, 187–188)

8   The lensmeter reads the distance portion of a lens prescription to be −1.50 sphere. When reading the bifocal add, the lensmeter drum reads +1.25. What is the strength of the bifocal add in this prescription?

    a. +1.25
    b. +1.00
    c. +2.75
    d. +2.00

ANSWER   **c.** +2.75

EXPLANATION   The total number of units traversed by the lensmeter power drum moving from −1.50 to +1.25 is 2.75. The drum moves from −1.50 to zero (a +1.50 change) and then moves to +1.25 for sharp focus of the mires (a +1.25 change). Therefore, +1.50 and +1.25 = +2.75. (Newmark 2006, 70, 72)

9   What is true about the intermediate segment in a trifocal lens?

    a. It is always half the power of the bifocal.
    b. It can be read with the PAL reader.
    c. It can be read using the lensmeter.
    d. It is twice the power of the bifocal add.

ANSWER   **c.** It can be read using the lensmeter.

EXPLANATION   The lensmeter can read the power of the intermediate segment of a trifocal lens. Although the intermediate power of most trifocals is half the power of the bifocal, it is not necessarily so; therefore, the intermediate power should be read separately. The PAL (progressive addition lens) reader device will allow you to read the add power engraved on the lens by the manufacturer but not the intermediate zone. (Newmark 2006, 70, 72)

10   The following occurs while taking a lensmeter reading: the single lines focus at –3.00; the triple lines focus at –4.50 with the axis at 055°. What would be the eyeglass prescription?

    a. –4.50 –3.00 axis 145
    b. –3.00 –4.50 axis 055
    c. –3.00 –2.50 axis 145
    d. –3.00 –1.50 axis 055

ANSWER   **d.** –3.00 –1.50 axis 055

EXPLANATION   The single lines focused at –3.00, so the sphere power is –3.00. The triple lines focused at –4.50; hence an additional –1.50 was needed over the –3.00 sphere. The axis on the cylinder axis wheel was 055°, so that is the axis for the –1.50 cylinder. All the other prescriptions are incorrect because in minus cylinder lensmeter readings the single lines focus on the sphere power and the triple lines focus on the cylinder only when the axis is set correctly on the cylinder axis wheel (in this case 055). The only calculation required is to subtract the sphere power reading from the cylinder power reading on the power drum to obtain the prescription cylinder power, which in this case was –1.50 (4.50 minus 3.00). (Newmark 2006, 72)

11   What maneuver should be performed before adjusting the eyepiece on the lensmeter to obtain the most accurate reading?

    a. Turn the eyepiece to reflect the axis of your astigmatism.
    b. Turn the eyepiece to the most minus position.
    c. Turn the eyepiece to the neutral position.
    d. Turn the eyepiece to the most plus position.

ANSWER   **d.** Turn the eyepiece to the most plus position.

EXPLANATION   Before adjusting the eyepiece, you should turn it to the most plus direction. This will fog (blur) the target seen through the eyepiece. Slowly turn the eyepiece toward the neutral position just until the target is clear, and then stop. The eyepiece has no astigmatic correction for the operator. One should use their usual corrective lenses when using the lensmeter. The most minus position may force the operator's eye to accommodate and the focus of the eyepiece will be erroneous. For some operators the neutral position may be the correct focus, however, to avoid erroneous readings the eyepiece adjustment must be verified each time the instrument is used. (Newmark 2006, 69–71)

12 During lensometry, what is the prism power and orientation of a right lens where the focused lines are displaced to the right and the lines cross at the second circle?

a. 4 prism diopters base down
b. 2 prism diopters base out
c. 2 prism diopters base in
d. 4 prism diopters base up

ANSWER c. 2 prism diopters base in

EXPLANATION The concentric circles in the target of a lensmeter will determine the power and orientation of a prism in an optical lens. The power is determined at the circle where the focused lines cross (in this case the second circle = 2 diopters). The crossed lines are displaced from the optical center (the lines will not center) and settle on a circle to the right, left, up, or down. When you are reading a left lens or right lens, up and down displacement is simply base up or base down in either eye. However, you must be mindful of which lens you are reading when determining base in or base out prism displacement. A right lens with displacement to the right has moved nasally or inward (base in) as in this case. However, a left lens with displacement to the right has moved temporally or outward (base out). The corollary is a right lens displaced left is base out and a left lens displaced left is base in. (Newmark 2006, 73)

5 KERATOMETRY

1 What is the method used to measure astigmatism?

a. A-scan ultrasound
b. ocular coherence tomography
c. lensometry
d. keratometry

ANSWER d. keratometry

EXPLANATION Keratometry is the method used to measure astigmatism. A-scan ultrasound is useful for measuring the axial length of the globe. Ocular coherence tomography (OCT) is used to create images of the macula and/or optic nerve. Lensometry is the measurement of certain qualities of lenses, such as the prescription of an eyeglass. (Newmark 2006, 73)

2   What is the first step in performing manual keratometry?

   a. Center the reticule in the bottom right circle.
   b. Focus the cross hairs.
   c. Align the axes.
   d. Fuse the plus signs and the minus signs.

ANSWER   **b.** Focus the cross hairs.

EXPLANATION   If the cross hairs (reticule) in the keratometer are not in focus, the dioptric powers of the cornea will not be accurately measured; therefore, using the eyepiece focusing of the cross hairs is the first step in performing keratometry. Centering the reticule, aligning the axes, and fusing the plus and minus signs are subsequent steps in performing manual keratometry. (Newmark 2006, 74–75)

3   What is an important step in performing keratometry?

   a. Occlude the eye not being measured.
   b. Keep both eyes looking through the machine.
   c. Occlude the eye being tested.
   d. Put the correct prism in the device for accurate measurements.

ANSWER   **a.** Occlude the eye not being measured.

EXPLANATION   When performing keratometry, it is important for the examiner to occlude the eye not being measured so that the measured eye is looking directly into the center of the keratometer barrel. Otherwise, the other eye may be fixating on the target, leading to inaccurate measurements. Prisms are not used in keratometry but rather in lensometry to measure the amount of prism in glasses. (Newmark 2006, 74)

4   The manual keratometer measures how much of the cornea?

   a. the whole corneal curvature
   b. approximately 3 mm of the center
   c. approximately 8 mm of the center
   d. the periphery and the center separately

ANSWER   **b.** approximately 3 mm of the center

EXPLANATION   The manual keratometer measures the central 3 mm of the cornea. The whole curvature is not measured by a manual device, nor is 8 mm of the center. Keratometry does not measure both the center and periphery, only the center. (Newmark 2006, 291)

5   What is the average corneal curvature of the human eye?

   a. 39.00 D
   b. 41.00 D

c. 43.00 D
d. 45.00 D

ANSWER   **c.** 43.00 D

EXPLANATION   The average corneal curvature (keratometry measurement) is 43.00 D. Corneal curvature measurements are part of the information needed to calculate intraocular lens implant power. These measurements are also used to fit contact lenses and are helpful in determining the astigmatic refractive error. (Kendall 1991, 161–162)

6   When the keratometer is properly aimed at the eye, how many circles will you see?

a. 1 circle
b. 2 circles
c. 3 circles
d. 4 circles

ANSWER   **c.** 3 circles

EXPLANATION   Three circles are found in the manual keratometer. The other answers are not correct. (Newmark 2006, 74–75)

7   Keratometry is useful for which of the following?

a. measuring the dioptric power of the cornea
b. determining the power of glasses
c. measuring the length of the eye
d. determining the health of the retina

ANSWER   **a.** measuring the dioptric power of the cornea

EXPLANATION   The keratometer measures the dioptric power (curvature) of the cornea. The measurement is important for lens implant calculations for cataract surgery. The lensmeter measures the power of eyeglass lenses. An A-scan ultrasound measures the length of the eye. The health of the retina can be determined by an ophthalmoscopic exam and automated methods, such as optical coherence tomography (OCT). (Newmark 2006, 17, 74–75)

8   What is the way to find the proper axis in keratometry?

a. Rotate the keratometer until a plus and minus sign align.
b. Dial the vertical scale knob until the reflection in the keratometer is greatest.
c. Rotate the keratometer until the 2 plus signs align.
d. Rotate the horizontal scale knob until the reflection is dimmest.

ANSWER   **c.** Rotate the keratometer until the 2 plus signs align.

EXPLANATION   The axis is measured by aligning the 2 plus signs. Overlapping the plus and minus signs would not give the correct axis. The vertical scale knob gives the power of the cornea in the vertical axis. The horizontal scale knob gives the power of the cornea in the horizontal axis. (Newmark 2006, 74–75)

9   Which of the following applies to keratometry in the fitting of contact lenses?
a. not useful because the fit is based on the power of the lens
b. useful because a good fit depends on corneal curvature
c. should be used only in hard contact lens fittings
d. does not work well when fitting soft lenses because it is too inaccurate

ANSWER   b. useful because a good fit depends upon corneal curvature

EXPLANATION   Contact lenses are fit well when they are measured based on the corneal curvature. The power of the lens is not a measurement for the fit of the contact, but for the refractive correction. Keratometry is useful in fitting both hard and soft contact lenses and is very accurate. (Newmark 2006, 73, 121)

10   Why is keratometry helpful in fitting contact lenses?
a. because the axis of the astigmatism is all that is needed
b. because it measures all of the parameters needed to fit a contact lens
c. because it measures the astigmatism to fit toric contact lenses exclusively
d. because a good fit requires both the axis and the amount of astigmatism

ANSWER   d. because a good fit requires both the axis and the amount of astigmatism.

EXPLANATION   When fitting contacts, a good fit is important and a keratometry measurement provides the axis and the amount of astigmatism on the cornea. Soft contact lenses that correct for astigmatism (toric lenses) can be more accurately selected when both parameters of the astigmatism are known. All contact lens fittings can benefit from keratometry readings, not just toric lenses. The corrective lens power of the eye is also needed to fit a contact lens. (Newmark 2006, 73–76, 195)

6 | MEDICAL ETHICS, LEGAL, AND REGULATORY ISSUES

1   One of the medical principals of ethics is that physicians should practice medicine primarily for the benefit of the patient. What is the primary responsibility of the ophthalmic medical assistant?
a. to work primarily for the benefit of the patient
b. to abide by state medical laws
c. to perform all tasks requested in an emergency
d. to treat the patient with respect, as the patient is always right

ANSWER   **b.** to abide by state medical laws

EXPLANATION   Ophthalmic medical assistants must abide by the laws of the state in which they function. Even in an emergency situation, they must function under the supervision of a licensed ophthalmologist or physician. The ophthalmologist's responsibility is to work primarily for the benefit of the patient but this requirement does not apply to assistants. Treating patients with respect is always advisable. However, patients may be confused or incorrectly report information and, therefore, are not always right. (Newmark 2006, 6–7)

2   Ethics are moral principles and values that govern individual behavior. Which of the following statements best applies to the professional code of ethics of the American Academy of Ophthalmology?

  a. The Code broadens the perspective of assistants.
  b. The Code requires physicians to set similar fees.
  c. The Code requires physicians to answer all patients' questions.
  d. The Code applies to all personnel on a member's staff.

ANSWER   **a.** The Code broadens the perspective of assistants.

EXPLANATION   The Academy's Code of Ethics states that fees for ophthalmologic services must not exploit patients or others but does not specify fees. The Code discusses general guidelines regarding care and respect of patients but does not address the issue of patient questions. The Academy's Code of Ethics applies to members of the Academy and does not strictly apply to a member's staff, although ophthalmic medical assistants will benefit from understanding the ethical principles and rules represented. (Newmark 2006, 7)

3   Which governing body recognizes JCAHPO certification and why?

  a. Federal and state governments recognize JCAHPO certification as part of hospital or clinic licensing requirements.
  b. The American Board of Specialty Boards recognizes JCAHPO certification to ensure oversight of medical assistants.
  c. Employers recognize JCAHPO certification as evidence of having achieved a certain level of competence.
  d. Some state medical boards recognize JCAHPO certification as sufficient for diagnosis but not treatment of some eye conditions.

ANSWER   **c.** Employers recognize JCAHPO certification as evidence of having achieved a certain level of competence.

EXPLANATION   JCAHPO certification attests to the skills and knowledge of individuals, indicating that they meet certain educational and experiential prerequisites and have passed an examination. JCAHPO certification is not required for state or federal hospital licensing. The American Board of Specialty Boards certifies physicians' competence and does not oversee medical assistants. State medical boards regulate physicians, dentists, and other professions, but not ophthalmic technical staff. Medical diagnosis requires licensure under a state medical or other professional board. (Newmark 2006, 4)

4   What does HIPAA protect?

  a. patient's privacy
  b. patient's finances
  c. patient's ability to decide the course of treatment
  d. patient's right for a second opinion

ANSWER   **a.** patient's privacy

EXPLANATION   The Health Insurance Portability and Accountability Act of 1996 (HIPAA) outlines very strict and specific rules about sharing patients' health information. (Newmark 2006, 7, 228, 277)

5   Under HIPAA (Health Insurance Portability and Accountability Act) regulations, the doctor may without permission disclose medical information to which of the patient's relationships?

  a. spouse
  b. child
  c. physician(s)
  d. attorney

ANSWER   **c.** physician(s)

EXPLANATION   The other physicians of the patient are the only exception to the requirement for a patient's permission to disclose health information or to provide medical care to the patient. It is important to talk to your office manager or supervisor to become knowledgeable about office policies and procedures regarding HIPAA patient privacy regulations. (Newmark 2006, 8)

6   Mrs. Smith's daughter calls the office to discuss her mother's medical condition. What should you do?

  a. Give her all the information she asked for.
  b. Ask for approval from Mrs. Smith to discuss her medical condition with her daughter.
  c. Do not discuss it but give her a copy of the record.
  d. Give her the diagnosis but no other information.

ANSWER   **b.** Ask for approval from Mrs. Smith to discuss her medical condition with her daughter.

EXPLANATION   Any patient's condition cannot be discussed with anyone, even a family member, without the patient's consent. The federal HIPAA law specifically forbids releasing confidential medical information without the patient's written permission. (Newmark 2006, 228)

7   You saw your neighbor in the office last week. If you reveal her medical information to her friends without her permission, which of the following would apply?

    a. You may be fined under state law.
    b. You may be jailed under HIPAA law.
    c. Your employer may be held responsible for a fine or criminal violation.
    d. All of the above apply.

ANSWER   **d.** All of the above apply.

EXPLANATION   Voluntary unauthorized disclosure of another's medical information risks potential civil legal penalties (fines or lawsuit) under state law and federal criminal penalties (jail time and/or fines under the Health Insurance Portability and Accountability Act of 1996). If your employer directed or participated in the disclosure, your employer may be found responsible as well. (Newmark 2006, 7, 288)

8   Why is informed consent important?

    a. It is necessary to have so that the physician is protected.
    b. It is necessary that the patient understands the procedure and its risks and benefits.
    c. It is required by the hospital.
    d. It is needed only for major surgery.

ANSWER   **b.** It is necessary that the patient understands the procedure and its risks and benefits.

EXPLANATION   Informed consent is necessary for any minor or major procedure performed on a patient. It does not protect the physician from malpractice action if malpractice has occurred. It is not done because it is required by the hospital, but because it is important that the patient be informed about the procedure and the risks and benefits of the surgery. (Newmark 2006, 244)

9   Which of the following best describes informed consent?

    a. It is a signature on the permission form.
    b. It is a protection for the surgeon.
    c. It is a protection for the clinic.
    d. It is a process.

ANSWER   **d.** It is a process.

EXPLANATION   Obtaining informed consent is known as the process of informing the patient about the risks, potential benefits, and alternatives of a proposed procedure or treatment. The process helps to protect patients by ensuring that they have received appropriate information and have given their permission for an intervention. Documentation of the process by the patient's or a legal guardian's signature serves as evidence that the process took place and may be used later to protect the physician from legal claims. (Newmark 2006, 244)

10   In obtaining valid informed consent, which of the following factors must be considered?

    a. native language of the patient
    b. IQ of the patient
    c. mood of the patient
    d. prior surgical experiences of the patient

ANSWER   **a.** native language of the patient

EXPLANATION   The native language of the patient must be considered in the process of obtaining consent. Proper consent assumes understanding by the patient, which may best be communicated in their native tongue. Other factors such as patient intellect, mood, and prior experiences may guide the ophthalmologist and their staff in completing pre-procedure discussions. (Newmark 2006, 244)

11   Which statement is correct regarding prescription medications?

    a. Many prescriptions may be called in to the pharmacy by the ophthalmic medical assistant.
    b. All prescriptions must include the doctor's license number.
    c. Prescriptions to be filled as needed must be undated.
    d. Only controlled substances such as narcotics require refill instructions.

ANSWER   **a.** Many prescriptions may be called in to the pharmacy by the ophthalmic medical assistant.

EXPLANATION   Many prescriptions can be called in to the pharmacy; controlled substances such as narcotics are an exception. The doctor's medical license number is required only for controlled substances. All prescriptions should be dated. Authorization or lack of authorization for refills can be noted on all prescriptions. (Newmark 2006, 89)

12   Which of the following responses applies to unauthorized removal of drugs or eyedrops from a medical office or hospital?

    a. This is allowed for temporary emergency treatment.
    b. This is unlawful and unethical.
    c. This is allowed to treat an indigent or self-pay patient.
    d. This triggers an investigation by the Drug Enforcement Administration (DEA).

ANSWER   **b.** This is unlawful and unethical.

EXPLANATION   Unauthorized removal of drugs or eyedrops from a medical office or hospital constitutes theft. If the drugs removed are among those regulated by the Drug Enforcement Administration (usually narcotics and hypnotics), the discovery of the unauthorized removal may trigger a federal administrative or criminal investigation. (Newmark 2006, 7)

13   If during history taking you suspect domestic abuse, what should you do?

    a. Call 911 or the local domestic abuse hotline.
    b. Talk to the ophthalmologist immediately.
    c. Document your interpretation in the medical record.
    d. Order x-rays to document hidden or old fractures.

ANSWER   **b.** Talk to the ophthalmologist immediately.

EXPLANATION   If you suspect domestic abuse, immediately discuss your concerns in private with the ophthalmologist. Other interventions should be performed only on the physician's expressed instruction. (Newmark 2006, 237)

14   If you are the first person to discover a fallen patient, what should you do?

    a. Assist the patient into a chair.
    b. Arrange for the patient's transportation to the emergency room.
    c. Start CPR.
    d. Notify the physician.

ANSWER   **d.** Notify the physician.

EXPLANATION   Your first responsibility is to notify the physician and call for help. After this, if the patient is unresponsive and has no pulse or respirations, then CPR should be initiated. One should not move the patient or allow the patient to leave the office until the physician has evaluated the injury. (Newmark 2006, 222)

15   The Centers for Disease Control (CDC) developed universal precautions to reduce transmission of which of the following?

    a. viruses (such as HIV)
    b. bacteria (such as methicillin-resistant *Staphylococcus aureus*)
    c. parasites (such as toxoplasmosis)
    d. prions (such as mad-cow disease)

ANSWER   **a.** viruses (such as HIV)

EXPLANATION   Universal precautions were developed by the CDC in response to the rise of the acquired immunodeficiency syndrome (AIDS) epidemic in the 1980s. AIDS is caused by several serotypes of human immunodeficiency virus (HIV). Although the guidelines were developed as a response to reduce transmission of and infection by HIV, they require medical workers to assume that all human blood and body fluids may be infectious, due to bloodborne pathogens such as viruses, bacteria, parasites, and other microbes. (Centers for Disease Control and Prevention 2009 [see Suggested Reading]; Newmark 2006, 102)

16   The Centers for Disease Control (CDC) has designated "body substance isolation precautions." Regarding these precautions, which of the following statements applies?

    a. They are mandated by OSHA (Occupational Safety & Health Administration).
    b. They are not included in "standard precautions."
    c. They apply to excimer laser exposure.
    d. They do not apply to tears, aqueous, and vitreous if uncontaminated by blood.

ANSWER   **c.** They apply to excimer laser exposure.

EXPLANATION   OSHA mandates the use of *universal precautions* only. *Standard precautions* combine the universal and body substance isolation precautions. These include precautions against bloodborne pathogens (universal precautions) as well as precautions for tears, aqueous, and vitreous. Precautions such as the use of masks and gloves to avoid potential transmission of infection from airborne droplets produced by excimer laser use are also included. (American Academy of Ophthalmology 2002 [see Suggested Reading]; Newmark 2006, 102–104)

17   Which of the following statements applies to universal precautions and hand washing?

    a. Hand washing is not required before wearing gloves.
    b. Hand washing is not required after wearing gloves.
    c. Hand washing with a germicide sterilizes the skin.
    d. Hand washing is required by OSHA.

ANSWER   **d.** Hand washing is required by OSHA.

EXPLANATION   Hand washing is an important part of universal infectious precautions and is mandated by OSHA to protect health care workers and patients. Hand washing should be performed before and after wearing gloves. Skin microbial concentrations ("counts") may be reduced substantially by application of a germicide but the skin should not be considered sterile. (Newmark 2006, 102–103)

18   Increasingly specific diagnoses can be coded using the ICD-9-CM system (International Classification of Diseases, ninth revision, clinical modification) by adding additional digits to a more general diagnosis code. Which of the following statements best characterizes ICD-9-CM coding?

    a. When a diagnosis is not known, no ICD-9-CM code should be applied.
    b. When a diagnosis is not known, a suspected diagnosis should be applied.
    c. Coding should be finalized to the highest level of specificity.
    d. A diagnosis cannot be a symptom.

ANSWER   **c.** Coding should be finalized to the highest level of specificity.

EXPLANATION   Diagnostic coding should be extended to include the most specific diagnosis known. If a diagnosis is not known, ICD-9-CM codes provided for symptoms and findings (such as eye pain) should be applied. (Newmark 2006, 278–279)

19   Which of the following statements applies to medical coding?

    a. Coding is the language of processing insurance claims.

    b. Coding is acceptable as documentation for service provided.

    c. Coding makes no distinction between diagnoses and procedures.

    d. Coding facilitates understanding of disease complexity.

ANSWER   **a.** Coding is the language of processing insurance claims.

EXPLANATION   Coding is the language of processing insurance claims and is not acceptable as documentation for service provided. Current Procedural Terminology (CPT) codes are the codes that indicate examinations and treatments. International Classification of Diseases, ninth revision, clinical modification (ICD-9-CM) provides codes for diagnoses. There is little ability within either of these coding systems to indicate disease severity or complexity. (Newmark 2006, 277–280)

20   Ophthalmic medical assistants are not allowed to practice independently of a physician; however, they may always perform which of the following?

    a. Diagnose a condition.

    b. Suggest a treatment.

    c. Estimate a prognosis.

    d. Provide an explanation of why and how a test will be performed.

ANSWER   **d.** Provide an explanation of why and how a test will be performed.

EXPLANATION   Ophthalmic medical assistants should never try to diagnose a condition, suggest treatments, or determine prognosis without the expressed instruction from an ophthalmologist to do so. Explaining how a test is performed or why it is ordered is important to elicit cooperation from the patient and is highly desirable. (Newmark 2006, 6–7)

21   Which of the following is **not** part of a proper informed consent?

    a. discussion of the disease or problem for which surgery is proposed

    b. an agreement not to sue the doctor

    c. discussion of the risks and benefits of the proposed surgery

    d. discussion of alternative treatments

ANSWER   **b.** an agreement not to sue the doctor

EXPLANATION   An informed consent involves a discussion with the patient, so that the patient can make an informed decision about whether to have a surgery performed. This includes the nature of the patient's problem, alternatives to surgery or alternative surgical procedures, and the potential risks and benefits of the proposed surgery, in comparison to the alternatives. An agreement not to sue would be considered coercive and would not protect the doctor in the event his or her negligence led to a significant surgical complication. (Newmark 2006, 244)

7 MICROBIOLOGY

1   Which of the following is a bacterium?
  a. herpes
  b. *Streptococcus*
  c. *Histoplasma*
  d. *Acanthamoeba*

ANSWER   **b.** *Streptococcus*

EXPLANATION   Bacteria are simple, single-celled microorganisms. *Streptococcus* is a Gram-positive bacterium. Herpes is a virus, *Histoplasma* is a fungus, and *Acanthamoeba* is a protozoan. (Newmark 2006, 96)

2   Contact lens wearers who use homemade solution to clean their lenses are most likely to develop a corneal infection caused by which type of organism?
  a. bacteria
  b. virus
  c. fungi
  d. protozoa

ANSWER   **d.** protozoa

EXPLANATION   The protozoan *Acanthamoeba* is a widespread organism in nonsterile water and is a likely cause of a contact lens-related corneal infection when homemade solutions are used. (Newmark 2006, 99–100)

3   What is the organism that is often associated with improper contact lens wear?
  a. *Staphylococcus aureus*
  b. *Pseudomonas aeruginosa*
  c. *Bacillus cereus*
  d. *Neisseria gonorrhoeae*

ANSWER   **b.** *Pseudomonas aeruginosa*

EXPLANATION   *Pseudomonas aeruginosa* is a Gram-negative organism that can contaminate eyedrops, contact lens cases, cosmetics, and hot tubs. *P aeruginosa* can cause serious corneal ulcers. *Staphylococcus aureus* is a Gram-positive organism and a frequent cause of blepharitis, conjunctivitis, and infectious keratitis. *Bacillus cereus* is also a Gram-positive organism, but it is a less common cause of ocular infections. *Neisseria gonorrhoeae* is a Gram-negative organism transmitted by sexual contact or congenital exposure in an infected birth canal, causing hyperacute conjunctivitis. (Newmark 2006, 97, 208)

4   Which statement is correct regarding ocular infections?

    a. Herpes simplex virus types I and II may cause ocular infections.

    b. Protozoa that cause ocular infections have very limited distribution in the environment.

    c. Treatment of fungal infections is shorter in duration and less difficult than treatment of bacterial infections.

    d. Varicella-zoster virus and adenovirus infections cause shingles.

ANSWER   **a.** Herpes simplex virus types I and II may cause ocular infections.

EXPLANATION   Herpes simplex virus types I and II may cause ocular infections. Protozoa are widely distributed in the environment, including soil and both salt and fresh water. The course of treatment for fungal infections is often quite extended compared to therapy for bacterial infections. Varicella-zoster virus causes chicken pox and shingles; adenovirus causes respiratory infections and conjunctivitis. (Newmark 2006, 98)

5   Which statement is correct regarding infection control precautions?

    a. Blood-soaked gauze should be placed in a rigid, puncture-proof biohazard container.

    b. Use of gloves to avoid contact with blood or body fluids makes hand washing unnecessary.

    c. Hand washing is one of the most important of the standard precautions.

    d. Universal precautions are used if blood has tested positive for pathogens.

ANSWER   **c.** Hand washing is one of the most important of the standard precautions.

EXPLANATION   Washing hands between patient contacts is the most important part of basic standard precautions. These precautions also include wearing disposable gloves, using "sharps" containers, proper disposal of contaminated objects, wearing a gown and mask when splashing of fluids is possible, and disposal of patches or gauze saturated with blood in a red bag. (CDC 2009 [see Suggested Reading]; Newmark 2006, 102–104)

6   Which statement is correct regarding disinfection?

    a. Disinfection may be accomplished with application of heat or chemicals.

    b. Disinfection takes longer than sterilization but more completely kills disease-causing microorganisms.

    c. Tonometer tips require no further disinfection if allowed to dry between patients.

    d. Cleaning equipment to remove organic material is not required if disinfection is performed immediately after use.

ANSWER   **a.** Disinfection may be accomplished with application of heat or chemicals.

EXPLANATION   Disinfection may be accomplished by heat (eg, boiling) or by germicidal chemicals. Disinfection eliminates most microbes, but only sterilization kills all living microorganisms.

Germicidal agents are always used for disinfection of tonometer tips. Cleaning and washing equipment to remove all organic material should be performed prior to disinfection or sterilization. (Newmark 2006, 104)

8 | PHARMACOLOGY

1   Which statement is correct regarding topical eye medication?

   a. Suspensions do not require a preservative.
   b. Solutions prevent systemic absorption.
   c. Properly administered ointments do not blur vision.
   d. Suspensions must be shaken vigorously before use.

ANSWER   **d.** Suspensions must be shaken vigorously before use.

EXPLANATION   Suspensions must be shaken vigorously before use. Most eyedrops, including suspensions, incorporate a preservative to inhibit the growth of bacteria or other organisms during storage. Eyedrop solutions drain from the eye through the lacrimal system and into the nose and throat and may be systemically absorbed. Ointments may blur vision due to their inherent physical properties. (Newmark 2006, 80)

2   The term *subcutaneous* refers to an injection that is given in what location?

   a. into the eye
   b. into a vein
   c. into a muscle
   d. under the skin

ANSWER   **d.** under the skin

EXPLANATION   *Subcutaneous* refers to an injection under the skin. An intravitreal injection is given into the eye, an intravenous injection is given into a vein, and an intramuscular injection is given into a muscle. (Newmark 2006, 81)

3   What is the act of dilating the pupil called?

   a. mydriasis
   b. cycloplegia
   c. pupilloplasty
   d. miosis

ANSWER   **a.** mydriasis

EXPLANATION   Mydriasis is the act of dilating the pupil, usually by an agent that directly stimulates the iris dilator muscle. Cycloplegia refers to paralyzing the ciliary muscle. These agents secondarily paralyze the iris sphincter muscle, causing passive dilation of the pupil. Pupilloplasty is a surgery on the iris. Miosis is constriction of the pupil. (Newmark 2006, 81)

4 When is dapiprazole 0.5% ophthalmic solution used?
  a. to dilate the pupil
  b. to reverse pupillary dilation
  c. to treat infection
  d. to reduce inflammation

ANSWER **b.** to reverse pupillary dilation

EXPLANATION Dapiprazole (Rev-Eyes) drops are used to reverse pupillary dilation. However, they do not reverse strong cycloplegic drops such as cyclopentolate. Mydriatics dilate the pupil. Antibiotics treat infection. Corticosteroids and nonsteroidal anti-inflammatory drugs (NSAIDs) reduce inflammation. (Newmark 2006, 81)

5 When administering a drop to a patient, where should the technician instruct the patient to look?
  a. Look up with the head tilted forward.
  b. Look up with the head tilted backward.
  c. Look down with the head tilted forward.
  d. Look down with the head tilted backward.

ANSWER **b.** Look up with the head tilted backward.

EXPLANATION Looking up with the head tilted backward maximizes drug delivery. (Newmark 2006, 82)

6 Which statement is correct regarding side effects of ophthalmic medications?
  a. Miotics may cause rapid pulse and dry mouth.
  b. Anesthetics prevent an allergic reaction by deadening a nerve.
  c. Cycloplegics may precipitate an attack of angle-closure glaucoma.
  d. Unlike systemic corticosteroid therapy, topical application does not cause cataracts.

ANSWER **c.** Cycloplegics may precipitate an attack of angle-closure glaucoma.

EXPLANATION Because cycloplegics dilate the pupil, an attack of angle-closure glaucoma may be precipitated in patients with a narrow anterior chamber angle. Cycloplegics may cause rapid pulse and dry mouth but miotics do not. Anesthetics can produce an allergic reaction. Topical corticosteroids can cause cataracts. (Newmark 2006, 83)

7   An ophthalmic assistant accidentally instills a drop of atropine 1% instead of tropicamide (Mydriacyl 1%) into a patient's eyes. What should the assistant do immediately?

a. Inform the patient that he will require sunglasses for 2 weeks.
b. Inform the patient that his eyes will be dilated for 2 weeks.
c. Inform the ophthalmologist.
d. Rinse the cul-de-sac with sterile saline.

ANSWER   c. Inform the ophthalmologist.

EXPLANATION   Only the ophthalmologist has the training and authority to discuss a maloccurrence with the patient. It is important to understand why the accident occurred and to institute changes to prevent another similar occurrence. The ophthalmic medical assistant should not provide any information to the patient without guidance from the ophthalmologist. Although it may be helpful to wash out the residual atropine from the cul-de-sac, it should not be undertaken without guidance from the ophthalmologist. (Newmark 2006, 83)

8   Which of the following medications may cause rapid pulse?

a. atropine
b. timolol
c. nepafenac
d. neomycin

ANSWER   a. atropine

EXPLANATION   Atropine and other cycloplegic medications can cause rapid pulse. Timolol, which is a beta-blocker used to treat glaucoma, slows the pulse. Nepafenac is a nonsteroidal anti-inflammatory agent. Neomycin is an antibiotic, and both have no affect on the pulse rate. (Newmark 2006, 83)

9   Which statement is correct regarding ophthalmic medications?

a. All cycloplegic eyedrops may cause stinging when administered topically.
b. Suspensions remain on the ocular surface longer than solutions by preventing nasolacrimal drainage.
c. Local injection of anesthetics prevents systemic toxicity.
d. Unlike administration by injection, ophthalmic dyes administered topically do not cause allergic reactions.

ANSWER   a. All cycloplegic eyedrops may cause stinging when administered topically.

EXPLANATION   All cycloplegic eyedrops may cause stinging when administered topically. Suspensions do not remain in contact with the eye surface for any longer period than solutions. Intravenous, intramuscular, and subcutaneous injections cause active drug to travel throughout the body's circulatory system and therefore, are more likely to cause systemic toxicity. Ophthalmic dyes when applied topically may also cause allergic reactions. (Newmark 2006, 83)

10   Before Goldmann applanation tonometry is performed, it is most appropriate to instill which type of eyedrop?

a. anesthetic
b. antimicrobial
c. cycloplegic
d. miotic

ANSWER   a. anesthetic

EXPLANATION   It is necessary to use a topical anesthetic drop to numb the eye before performing tonometry, because the tonometer tip contacts the ocular surface. Antimicrobial, cycloplegic, and miotic drops are not anesthetics. An antimicrobial agent acts to kill or inhibit the growth of microorganisms. A cycloplegic agent inhibits accommodation and dilates the pupil. A miotic agent constricts the pupil. (Newmark 2006, 84, 130)

11   In a healthy eye, fluorescein dye should cause fluorescence (a bright yellow-green color under cobalt blue lighting) only of which one of the following?

a. tear film
b. conjunctiva
c. cornea
d. iris

ANSWER   a. tear film

EXPLANATION   In the normal eye, only the tear layer fluoresces, a characteristic that makes the dye useful for applanation tonometry and contact lens fitting. Fluorescein will also stain defective or absent corneal epithelium. (Newmark 2006, 84)

12   What dye is injected intravenously before angiography to highlight the retinal vessels?

a. lissamine green
b. fluorescein
c. rose bengal
d. gentian violet

ANSWER   b. fluorescein

EXPLANATION   Fluorescein angiography is the method used to highlight retinal vessels. Lissamine green, rose bengal, and topical fluorescein are dyes used to detect surface defects on the eye. Gentian violet is used as a surgical marker. (Newmark 2006, 84)

13   Which of the following is an anesthetic?

a. proparacaine (Alcaine)
b. pilocarpine (Isopto-Carpine)
c. travoprost (Travatan)
d. mannitol (Osmitrol)

ANSWER   **a.** proparacaine (Alcaine)

EXPLANATION   Proparacaine, an anesthetic, is sold under brand names including Alcaine, Ophthetic, and Ophthaine. Pilocarpine and travoprost are topical anti-glaucomatous medications, and mannitol is an intravenous medication for lowering intraocular pressure. (Newmark 2006, 84)

14   Brow ache, myopia, and retinal detachment are possible side effects of what type of medication?

    a. miotics
    b. cycloplegics
    c. carbonic anhydrase inhibitors
    d. prostaglandin analogs

ANSWER   **a.** miotics

EXPLANATION   Miotics can cause brow ache, myopia, and retinal attachments. In addition, miotics can cause increased tearing, sweating, salivation, and diarrhea. Cycloplegics can cause blurry vision and increased pulse rate. Carbonic anhydrase inhibitors can cause tingling in the extremities and metallic taste in the mouth. Prostaglandin analogs can increase pigmentation of the iris and eyelid skin as well as increase the length of the eyelashes. (Newmark 2006, 85)

15   If a patient reports a history of severe allergy to fluoroquinolones, what ophthalmic medicine might be dangerous for the patient?

    a. tobramycin drops
    b. ciprofloxacin drops
    c. timolol maleate drops
    d. acetazolamide tablets

ANSWER   **b.** ciprofloxacin drops

EXPLANATION   Patients who report an allergic reaction in the past to a medication should be questioned about the severity of the reaction (rash, breathing difficulties, cardiac arrest) and if they are allergic to any other medications. Of the medications listed, only ciprofloxacin drops are related to fluoroquinolones. These drops should be used with caution in a patient who reports a prior severe allergic reaction to that family of medications. Tobramycin is an antibiotic from a chemical family called *aminoglycosides*. Timolol is a beta-blocker agent and is used to treat glaucoma. Acetazolamide is a carbonic anhydrase inhibitor agent related to sulfonamides, and it is used orally to treat glaucoma. (Newmark 2006, 85–86)

16   Which statement is correct regarding antimicrobial therapy?

    a. So-called "fortified" antibiotics are available without a prescription.
    b. Topical antibiotics inhibit bacterial growth but systemic antibiotics kill bacteria.

c. Single antifungal or antiviral agents are widely used as a preventive measure.
d. Antivirals inhibit the ability of viruses to reproduce.

ANSWER   d. Antivirals inhibit the ability of viruses to reproduce.

EXPLANATION   Antiviral agents interfere with viral replication (the ability to reproduce). Fortified antibiotics are mixed by a pharmacist according to a physician's prescription. Topical antibiotics may inhibit or kill bacteria. Single antifungal and antiviral agents are used when the diagnosis is definitive or highly suspicious of the disease. (Newmark 2006, 86)

17   A patient has a flare-up of iritis. What is the most appropriate topical medication for treating this problem?

a. proparacaine ophthalmic solution
b. cyclosporine A emulsion
c. prednisolone acetate 1% suspension
d. timolol 1% solution

ANSWER   c. prednisolone acetate 1% suspension

EXPLANATION   Prednisolone acetate 1% suspension is a cortisone eyedrop having anti-inflammatory properties. This class of medication is commonly used to treat iritis. Proparacaine is a topical anesthetic used to anesthetize the surface of the eye. Cyclosporine A emulsion is a treatment for dry eyes, and timolol is a beta-blocker used as a treatment for glaucoma. (Newmark 2006, 37–38, 87)

18   Corticosteroids can cause which of the following?

a. cataract
b. lower intraocular pressure
c. encourage faster healing
d. increase growth of eye muscles

ANSWER   a. cataract

EXPLANATION   Corticosteroids in all forms of administration can cause cataracts, elevate intraocular pressure, and slow healing but do not increase the growth of eye muscles. In addition, corticosteroids can aggravate diseases such as systemic hypertension, diabetes mellitus, peptic ulcer, tuberculosis, and infection. (Newmark 2006, 87)

19   Cyclosporine A (Restasis) is a topical emulsification used in the treatment of what condition?

a. allergy
b. uveitis
c. tear deficiency
d. glaucoma

ANSWER   **c.** tear deficiency

EXPLANATION   Cyclosporine A (Restasis), although used off-label for some other purposes, is approved for the treatment of tear deficiency associated with autoimmune or inflammatory conditions of the eyelids. Cyclosporine A has no effect in lowering intraocular pressure to treat glaucoma. Although ocular allergy and uveitis are autoimmune inflammatory conditions, it is not FDA-approved for these conditions. (Newmark 2006, 88)

20   Mast-cell stabilizers, such as cromolyn (Crolom), are useful in the treatment of which one of the following?

   a. bacterial infection
   b. seasonal allergic conjunctivitis
   c. intraocular inflammation
   d. glaucoma

ANSWER   **b.** seasonal allergic conjunctivitis

EXPLANATION   Mast-cell stabilizers reduce the itching, tearing, and conjunctival injection associated with seasonal allergic conjunctivitis, generally seen in the spring and late summer months. Bacterial infections are treated with antibiotics. Intraocular inflammation not caused by microorganisms is treated with corticosteroids. Glaucoma is treated with drugs that reduce the intraocular pressure. (Newmark 2006, 88)

21   If a medication is written to be taken prn, when should it be taken?

   a. before meals
   b. before bedtime
   c. with food
   d. as needed

ANSWER   **d.** as needed

EXPLANATION   *Pro re nata*, or prn, refers to taking the medication as necessary. The abbreviations for instructions to take medications before meals, before bedtime, and with food are ac, hs, and cc respectively. (Newmark 2006, 89)

22   If the doctor's prescription indicates the abbreviation qid, how often should the medication be administered?

   a. once a day
   b. every hour
   c. 4 times a day
   d. every 4 hours

ANSWER   **c.** 4 times a day

EXPLANATION   The abbreviation qid comes from the Latin *quater in die*, meaning 4 times a day. Abbreviations for once a day, every hour, and every 4 hours are qd, q1h, and q4h respectively. (Newmark 2006, 89)

23   The abbreviation tid refers to a medication that is to be administered how often?

    a. every 3 hours
    b. 3 times a day
    c. every 4 hours
    d. 4 times a day

ANSWER   **b.** 3 times a day

EXPLANATION   The abbreviation tid is derived from the Latin *ter in die*, or 3 times a day. Four times a day would be written as qid. Every 3 hours is q3h and every 4 hours is q4h. (Newmark 2006, 89)

24   Which of the following is an acute drug reaction?

    a. fainting
    b. headache
    c. salty taste in mouth
    d. sneezing

ANSWER   **a.** fainting

EXPLANATION   Fainting is an acute drug reaction and should prompt a quick response. Sneezing, a rash, headache, dizziness are common other drug reactions, but are not acute in nature and do not require a prompt response. (Newmark 2006, 90)

25   Medications that may impair the blood-clotting mechanism are important to know about before surgery. These medications include which of the following?

    a. aspirin
    b. acetaminophen
    c. morphine
    d. codeine

ANSWER   **a.** aspirin

EXPLANATION   Many medicines and some supplements impair blood-clotting mechanisms, including aspirin, ibuprofen, ginkgo biloba, Vitamin E, ginseng, and others. Acetaminophen and morphine and morphine derivatives like codeine have no effect on clotting. Failure to elicit this information prior to surgery can result in serious bleeding complications. (Newmark 2006, 116)

26 Which of the following statements is accurate?

    a. Topical decongestants remove the cause of ocular irritation.
    b. Topical and systemic corticosteroid therapies may cause glaucoma and cataracts.
    c. Mast-cell stabilizers maintain an appropriate tear film balance.
    d. Preservative-free lubricants do not cause side effects.

ANSWER   **b.** Topical and systemic corticosteroid therapies may cause glaucoma and cataracts.

EXPLANATION   Chronic topical and systemic corticosteroid therapies may promote cataract and glaucoma as well as cause other unwanted effects. A topical decongestant acts by constricting superficial blood vessels in the conjunctiva but does not remove the cause of the dilated vessels. Mast-cell stabilizers reduce conjunctival allergic reactions. The lack of preservatives in lubricants reduces the likelihood of side effects, but does not entirely eliminate them. (Newmark 2006, 87)

27 Decongestants such as Visine can cause all **except** which one of the following?

    a. allergy
    b. angle-closure glaucoma
    c. rebound redness
    d. elevated blood sugar

ANSWER   **d.** elevated blood sugar

EXPLANATION   Elevated blood sugar is not a known side effect of decongestants. Decongestants contain vasoconstrictors (agents that narrow blood vessels), and have a tendency toward side effects such as the first 3 choices listed above. (Newmark 2006, 87)

28 The principal uses of a cycloplegic agent include all **except** which of the following?

    a. performing a refraction that requires an absence of accommodation
    b. decreasing a ciliary muscle spasm present in patients with uveitis
    c. conducting a fundus examination
    d. treating open-angle glaucoma

ANSWER   **d.** treating open-angle glaucoma

EXPLANATION   Cycloplegics are not used to treat open-angle glaucoma. (Newmark 2006, 83–84)

29 Which injection type is **not** classified as systemic drug delivery?

    a. intravitreal injection
    b. intravenous injection
    c. intramuscular injection
    d. subcutaneous injection

ANSWER   **a.** intravitreal injection

EXPLANATION   Intravitreal injection delivers active drug directly into the eye. The other choices involve active drug traveling through the circulatory system before reaching the eye. (Newmark 2006, 81)

30   Which of the following dye–color matches is **incorrect**?

    a. lissamine green – green
    b. rose bengal – rose
    c. fluorescein – yellow/green
    d. gentian violet – purple

ANSWER   **b.** rose bengal – rose

EXPLANATION   Rose bengal is a red dye. (Newmark 2006, 84)

31   Which of the following glaucoma medications is **not** a beta-adrenergic-blocker?

    a. timolol (Timoptic, Betimol)
    b. levobunolol (Betagan)
    c. mannitol (Osmitrol)
    d. carteolol (Ocupress)

ANSWER   **c.** mannitol (Osmitrol)

EXPLANATION   Mannitol is a hyperosmotic injectable agent with a variety of uses, including treatment of acute glaucoma. Hint: the –olol ending is often indicative of a beta-blocker medication. (Newmark 2006, 85)

32   Which of the following is **not** a nonsteroidal anti-inflammatory drug (NSAID)?

    a. diclofenac (Voltaren)
    b. flurbiprofen (Ocufen)
    c. loteprednol etabonate (Lotemax)
    d. bromfenac (Xibrom)

ANSWER   **c.** loteprednol etabonate (Lotemax)

EXPLANATION   Loteprednol is a corticosteroid and not a NSAID. To help you remember the NSAIDs from other eye medications, look at the suffix of the chemical name; they end either in "fen" or in "nac." (Newmark 2006, 87)

9 OCULAR MOTILITY

1   What is an outward deviation of the eye called?

a. exo deviation
b. eso deviation
c. hyper deviation
d. hypo deviation

ANSWER   a. exo deviation

EXPLANATION   Strabismus (figure) may be classified by the direction of the misalignment. Outward deviation of the eye is an exo deviation, inward deviation is an eso deviation, upward deviation is a hyper deviation, and downward deviation is a hypo deviation. (Newmark 2006, 31)

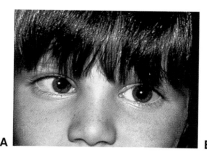 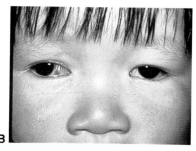

Stabismus. (A) Esotropia (eso deviation). Right eye is turned inward (light reflex is at the temporal corneal margin). (B) Exotropia (exo deviation). Right eye is turned outward (light reflex is at the nasal corneal margin). (Reproduced, with permission, from Newmark E, ed. *Ophthalmic Medical Assisting: An Independent Study Course*, 4th ed. American Academy of Ophthalmology, 2006.)

2   What combination of extraocular muscle actions occur when a patient looks to her left?

a. left lateral rectus contracts; right lateral rectus relaxes
b. left lateral rectus contracts; right lateral rectus contracts
c. left medial rectus contracts; right lateral rectus relaxes
d. left medial rectus relaxes; right medial rectus relaxes

ANSWER   a. left lateral rectus contracts; right lateral rectus relaxes

EXPLANATION   The figure illustrates the functions of the lateral and medial rectus muscles of the eye. In left gaze, the left lateral rectus and right medial rectus muscles contract, and the left medial rectus and right lateral rectus muscles relax. In right gaze, the right lateral rectus and left medial rectus muscles contract, and the right medial rectus and left lateral rectus muscles relax. (Newmark 2006, 13)

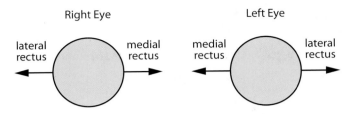

Lateral and medial rectus muscles of the eye.

3   What is tested when the cardinal positions of gaze are evaluated?

a. convergence
b. divergence
c. fusion
d. function of the 6 extraocular muscles

ANSWER   **d.** function of the 6 extraocular muscles

EXPLANATION   Evaluation of a patient's eye movements in the cardinal positions of gaze consists of: (1) right and up; (2) right; (3) right and down; (4) left and up; (5) left; and (6) left and down. These positions test the function of the 6 extraocular muscles (figure). Convergence and divergence movements use only a couple of specific muscles. Fusion is evaluated with the Worth 4-dot test. (Newmark 2006, 122)

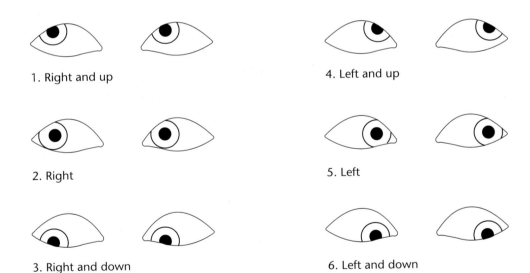

1. Right and up

4. Left and up

2. Right

5. Left

3. Right and down

6. Left and down

The 6 cardinal positions of gaze used to evaluate eye movement. (Reproduced, with permission, from Newmark E, ed. *Ophthalmic Medical Assisting: An Independent Study Course,* 4th ed. San Francisco: American Academy of Ophthalmology, 2006.)

4   When performing the cover-uncover test, the examiner notices that the uncovered eye moves in order to fix on the target. What does this probably represent?

a. tropia
b. suppression
c. phoria
d. amblyopia

ANSWER   **a.** tropia

EXPLANATION   If the *uncovered* eye moves while the cover-uncover test is being performed, it is an indication of a tropia. If the *covered* eye moves when the cover is removed, it is an indication of a phoria. Suppression may be evaluated by the Worth 4-dot test. Amblyopia is assessed by visual acuity testing. (Newmark 2006, 123)

5   The size of an ocular deviation may be measured by which of the following?
   a. prism and alternate cover test
   b. Worth 4-dot test
   c. Titmus fly
   d. exophthalmometer

ANSWER   **a.** prism and alternate cover test

EXPLANATION   An ocular deviation may be measured using the prism and alternate cover test (figure). The Worth 4-dot test measures fusion. The Titmus fly test measures depth perception (stereopsis). The exophthalmometer measures the prominence (bulging) of the eyeball in relation to the bony orbital rim. (Newmark 2006, 123)

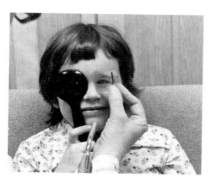

The prism and alternate cover test. (Reproduced, with permission, from Newmark E, ed. *Ophthalmic Medical Assisting: An Independent Study Course*, 4th ed. San Francisco: American Academy of Ophthalmology, 2006.)

6   During the cover-uncover test, neither eye moves when the cover is removed. This probably represents which of the following?
   a. tropia
   b. suppression
   c. orthophoria
   d. amblyopia

ANSWER   **c.** orthophoria

EXPLANATION   If neither eye moves when the cover is removed, it is an indication of normal alignment, or orthophoria. If the *covered* eye moves when the cover is removed, it is an indication of a phoria. If the *uncovered* eye moves in order to fix on the target, it is an indication of a tropia. Suppression may be evaluated by the Worth 4-dot test. Amblyopia is assessed by visual acuity testing. (Newmark 2006, 123, 180)

10 IN-OFFICE MINOR SURGICAL PROCEDURES

1   Prior to the patient's procedure, what is the assistant's major responsibility?

   a. Answer questions about the procedure.
   b. Put the patient at ease.
   c. Discuss the surgeon's ability to do the procedure.
   d. Discuss the disease process.

ANSWER   **b.** Put the patient at ease.

EXPLANATION   Before any procedure, the assistant's major responsibility is to put the patient at ease and make the visit as comfortable as possible. Topics to avoid include the surgeon's ability to do the procedure, previous outcomes, the disease condition itself, and risks of the treatment. If patients ask questions in these areas, they should be directed to the surgeon. (Newmark 2006, 244–245)

2   During minor office procedures, anesthesia often consists of which of the following?

   a. topical drops or locally injected anesthetic agents
   b. general inhalation anesthesia
   c. intravenous sedation
   d. tranquilizer

ANSWER   **a.** topical drops or locally injected anesthetic agents

EXPLANATION   Topical eyedrops (proparacaine, tetracaine, and lidocaine) and injectable anesthetics (often lidocaine) are the most commonly used office anesthetics. The addition of epinephrine to injectable lidocaine decreases bleeding and prolongs the effect of the anesthetic. General anesthesia and intravenous (IV) sedation are not utilized for minor in-office surgical procedures. Although a tranquilizer drug would relax the patient and make him or her more comfortable, it does not provide pain relief. (Newmark 2006, 245)

3   Which of the following is an instrument used to grasp tissue?

   a. scissors
   b. needle holder
   c. cannula
   d. forceps

ANSWER   **d.** forceps

EXPLANATION   Forceps, which are basically tweezers, are used to grasp tissue or sutures. Scissors are used to cut tissue or suture. A needle holder grasps a needle and helps drive it through the tissue. A cannula is basically a hollow blunt-ended needle used to inject or irrigate a fluid. (Newmark 2006, 246–247)

4   What instrument is used to stop bleeding?

   a. forceps
   b. cannula
   c. clamp
   d. needle

ANSWER   **c.** clamp

EXPLANATION   A clamp can be used to provide pressure to stop bleeding. A cannula is a blunt-ended needle used to inject or irrigate. A needle is used to suture tissue together. A forceps is used to grasp tissue. (Newmark 2006, 247)

5   What common minor surgical procedure is performed in the exam lane?

   a. cataract surgery
   b. ptosis repair
   c. trabeculectomy
   d. epilation

ANSWER   **d.** epilation

EXPLANATION   Cataract surgery, ptosis repair for a droopy eyelid, and trabeculectomy to relieve intraocular pressure are all done in an operating room. Epilation, or removal of in-growing eyelashes, can be done in the exam room at the slit lamp with a forceps. (Newmark 2006, 249–250)

6   Which phrase applies to the insertion of punctual plugs?

   a. requires an anesthetic injection
   b. is a method of managing dry eyes
   c. is a cure for dry eyes
   d. is painful

ANSWER   **b.** is a method of managing dry eyes

EXPLANATION   The insertion of punctual plugs is one of several methods to reduce dry eye symptoms. It requires only topical anesthesia and is rarely painful. Plugs are not a cure for dry eyes because ocular lubrication of the surface of the eye may still be inadequate and the plugs may fall out. (Newmark 2006, 251)

7   Which of the following patients is a poor candidate for LASIK?

   a. a patient with myopic astigmatism
   b. a patient with hyperopic astigmatism
   c. a patient with a normal but thick cornea
   d. a patient with a normal but thin cornea

ANSWER   **d.** a patient with a normal but thin cornea

EXPLANATION   LASIK surgery involves cutting across the anterior cornea, raising a flap of tissue, and removing a thin layer of tissue under the flap by using a laser. If the cornea is thin before surgery, removing tissue can leave the cornea abnormally thin with subsequent bulging (ectasia) postoperatively, leading to vision problems. Patients with myopic astigmatism, hyperopic astigmatism, or a normal but thick cornea may be good candidates for LASIK. (Newmark 2006, 262–264)

8   Which statement applies to refractive surgery?

    a. It is a minor procedure with minimal risks.
    b. It almost always results in the elimination of the need for glasses or contact lenses for the patient's lifetime.
    c. It is performed only with a laser.
    d. It often results in a decreased need for glasses or contact lenses.

ANSWER   **d.** It often results in a decreased need for glasses or contact lenses.

EXPLANATION   Although complications from refractive surgery are infrequent, they can be very serious. The result of refractive surgery frequently reduces the need for glasses or contact lenses; however, the surgery rarely eliminates their use for a lifetime because presbyopia, the aging eye's inability to focus on very near objects, is not eliminated. Most refractive procedures are performed with a laser, but incisional keratotomy, particularly for the reduction of astigmatism, is still widely practiced. (Newmark 2006, 262)

9   What type of refractive *intraocular* surgery, although controversial, is currently being performed?

    a. LASIK and LASEK
    b. phakic intraocular lenses
    c. photorefractive Keratectomy (PRK)
    d. astigmatic Keratotomy (AK)

ANSWER   **b.** phakic intraocular lenses

EXPLANATION   Only phakic intraocular lenses require intraocular surgery. All of the other procedures are performed on the surface of the eye. (Newmark 2006, 268)

10   During a surgical procedure that does not involve general sedation, how can the assistant best help the surgeon?

    a. by remaining very quiet
    b. by talking to the patient for reassurance
    c. by anticipating the surgeon's next step
    d. by preparing the surgical site

ANSWER   **c.** by anticipating the surgeon's next step

EXPLANATION   The assistant can help best during surgery by anticipating the next step and having the next instrument ready for the surgery or the cotton tip ready for blotting blood. Although superfluous chatter is not good in the operating room, it is not obligatory for the assistant to remain silent. During a surgical procedure where the patient remains awake, the patient must not move. Talking involves mouth movement, which in turn causes the eye to move, so it is best for the assistant not to speak to the patient directly during the surgery. Preparing the surgical site by prepping the area with antiseptic is done prior to surgery. (Newmark 2006, 257)

11   An ophthalmologist usually performs surgery in all **except** which of the following sites?

    a. operating room
    b. office exam lanes
    c. minor operating room
    d. patient's home

ANSWER   **d.** patient's home

EXPLANATION   An ophthalmologist usually performs surgery in an ambulatory or hospital operating room, in the exam lane, and in an in-office minor operating room. The patient's general health and the complexity of the case determine which setting will be used for the patient's surgery. The patient's home would not be a usual site to perform surgery. (Newmark 2006, 243)

12   Many minor surgical procedures can be performed in the ophthalmologist's office. They all have certain aspects in common **except** which of the following?

    a. explaining the purpose of the procedure and obtaining the patient's consent
    b. preparing the instruments and supplies
    c. assisting the ophthalmologist during the procedure
    d. having the patient call the ophthalmologist

ANSWER   **d.** having the patient call the ophthalmologist

EXPLANATION   Obtaining informed consent and explaining the procedure are primarily important before commencing any surgery. Preparing the instruments and supplies and assisting the surgeon then follow. Directing the patient to call the ophthalmologist is not part of the minor surgical procedure. (Newmark 2006, 244–245).

13   The sterile operating field includes all **except** which of the following?

    a. surgical gowns
    b. instrument tray
    c. protective eyewear
    d. drapes

ANSWER   **c.** protective eyewear

EXPLANATION   Although protective eyewear is important when using lasers or during open surgery, it is not part of the aseptic area and is not considered part of the operating field. (Newmark 2006, 255)

14   What instrument is **not** typically a part of a chalazion surgical set?

 a. scalpel blade and handle
 b. micro scissors
 c. curette
 d. needle holder

ANSWER   **d.** needle holder

EXPLANATION   A chronic chalazion is a nontender lump resulting from an obstructed meibomian gland in the eyelid. A needle holder is used to place sutures, which are generally not used during incision and drainage of a chalazion. A scalpel blade and handle, micro scissors, and a curette are instruments used for incising and draining a chalazion from an everted eyelid. (Newmark 2006, 250)

15   Which injection type is **not** classified as systemic drug delivery?

 a. intravitreal injection
 b. intravenous injection
 c. intramuscular injection
 d. subcutaneous injection

ANSWER   **a.** intravitreal injection

EXPLANATION   Intravitreal injection delivers active drug directly into the eye. The other choices involve active drug traveling through the circulatory system before reaching the eye. (Newmark 2006, 81)

16   Which of the following items is **not** considered part of the sterile field?

 a. the prepped part of the patient's body covered by a sterile drape
 b. the tables and trays covered with a sterile drape and the sterile instruments
 c. the surgical personnel, gowned and gloved
 d. the chest, arms, and hands of the patient

ANSWER   **d.** the chest, arms, and hands of the patient

EXPLANATION   For the patient, only the part of the patient's body that has been prepped and draped is in the sterile field. For the surgical personnel, the back and the part of the body above the chest and below the waist are not considered sterile. All tables and trays covered with sterile drapes and all sterile operating instruments are part of the sterile field. (Newmark 2006, 255)

11 OPHTHALMIC PATIENT SERVICES AND EDUCATION

1   In the following list, which is the best pairing?

    a. optician: diagnosis of optical problems
    b. ophthalmic assistant: removal of turned-in lashes
    c. optometrist: LASIK surgery
    d. ophthalmologist: informed consent process

ANSWER   **d.** ophthalmologist: informed consent process

EXPLANATION   The ophthalmologist is responsible for educating the patient about alternative choices, explaining risks and benefits, and answering questions before a patient can decide to have elective surgery. An optician fits corrective lenses according to the prescription of an ophthalmologist or optometrist. An optician is not licensed or certified to diagnose optical problems. An ophthalmic medical assistant is not responsible for treating eye diseases, and optometrists are not licensed to perform LASIK surgery. (Newmark 2006, 2–4)

2   What is a wedge-shaped growth of conjunctival tissue that grows onto the cornea?

    a. chalazion
    b. pinguecula
    c. nevus
    d. pterygium

ANSWER   **d.** pterygium

EXPLANATION   The correct answer is pterygium (figure). A pterygium is wedge or wing-shaped, hence its name, which is derived from the Greek root, *ptery*, for wing. A chalazion is a granulomatous inflammation of a meibomian gland in the eyelid. A nevus is a benign, pigmented growth, which is a form of a freckle. A pinguecula is a mass of degenerated conjunctival tissue that is similar to a pterygium, but does not grow onto the cornea. (Newmark 2006, 35)

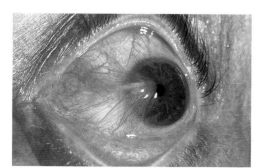

Conjunctival disorders. Pterygium. (Reproduced, with permission, from Newmark E, ed. *Ophthalmic Medical Assisting: An Independent Study Course,* 4th ed. San Francisco: American Academy of Ophthalmology; 2006.)

3   What is the medical term for blood in the anterior chamber?

    a. rubeosis iridis
    b. hypopyon
    c. blunt trauma
    d. hyphema

ANSWER   **d.** hyphema

EXPLANATION   Blood in the anterior chamber is called a hyphema (figure) Rubeosis iridis, or abnormal blood vessels on the iris, may leak and cause bleeding into the anterior chamber. Hypopyon is a layer of white blood cells (pus) in the anterior chamber and is a sign of serious internal ocular inflammation or infection. Blunt trauma may result in bleeding in the anterior chamber. (Newmark 2006, 36)

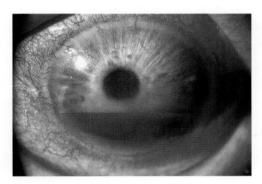

Hyphema. Note blood layer in anterior chamber obscuring iris structure. (Reproduced, with permission, from Newmark E, ed. *Ophthalmic Medical Assisting: An Independent Study Course,* 4th ed. San Francisco: American Academy of Ophthalmology; 2006.)

4   What is the term for a turning in of the lower eyelid margin?

    a. ectropion
    b. ptosis
    c. trichiasis
    d. entropion

ANSWER   **d.** entropion

EXPLANATION   Entropion is an inturning of the eyelid margin. Ectropion is a turning out of the eyelid margin, and ptosis is a drooping eyelid. Trichiasis is inturned lashes, which may or may not occur with entropion. (Newmark 2006, 15, 33)

5   Which of the following is found in the conjunctiva?

    a. goblet cells
    b. meibomian glands
    c. lacrimal sac
    d. cilia

ANSWER   **a.** goblet cells

EXPLANATION   Goblet cells are specific cells in the conjunctiva that produce mucinous (sticky) fluid as part of the tear film. Meibomian glands are oil glands in the eyelid, the lacrimal sac is the part of the tear drainage system between the canaliculus and the nasolacrimal duct, and cilia are the eyelashes. (Newmark 2006, 16)

6   What is the condition referring to inflammation of the lacrimal sac?

    a. canaliculitis
    b. dacryoadenitis
    c. trichiasis
    d. dacryocystitis

ANSWER   **d.** dacryocystitis

EXPLANATION   Dacryocystitis is an inflammation of the lacrimal sac (figure). Dacryoadenitis is an inflammation of the lacrimal gland, canaliculitis is an inflammation of the canaliculus, and trichiasis is the inward misdirection of eyelashes. (Newmark 2006, 17, 33)

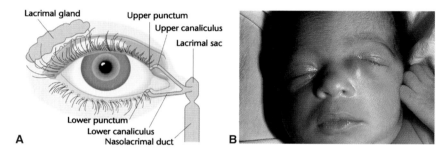

Anatomic drawing of the lacrimal apparatus (A) and example of dacryocystitis (B). (Reproduced, with permission, from Newmark E, ed. *Ophthalmic Medical Assisting: An Independent Study Course*, 4th ed. San Francisco: American Academy of Ophthalmology; 2006.)

7   The anterior chamber angle is formed by the junction of which structures?

    a. ciliary body and lens zonules
    b. cornea and sclera
    c. cornea and iris
    d. anterior and posterior chamber

ANSWER   **c.** cornea and iris

EXPLANATION   The anterior chamber angle (figure) is the location of the trabecular meshwork and Schlemm's canal, which is the area that controls the drainage of aqueous humor from the eye and thereby controls intraocular pressure. It forms an angle where the iris and cornea meet. The junction of the cornea and sclera is called the *limbus*. Zonules originate from the ciliary body and do not form an angle. The anterior and posterior chambers are connected by the pupil and separated by the iris and do not form an angle. (Newmark 2006, 18)

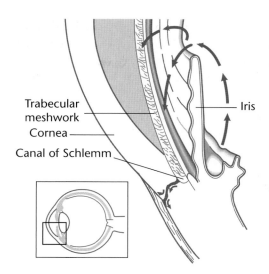

The anterior chamber angle and the flow of aqueous fluid (Reproduced, with permission, from Newmark E, ed. *Ophthalmic Medical Assisting: An Independent Study Course,* 4th ed. San Francisco: American Academy of Ophthalmology; 2006.)

8   Where are floaters found?

  a. aqueous humor
  b. lens
  c. vitreous
  d. retina

ANSWER   **c.** vitreous

EXPLANATION   Floaters are particles in the vitreous. (Newmark 2006, 20)

9   Through which structures does light pass before reaching the photoreceptors (rods and cones)?

  a. ganglion cells
  b. retinal pigment epithelium
  c. ciliary body
  d. choroid

ANSWER   **a.** ganglion cells

EXPLANATION   Light passes through a number of structures, fluid- and tissue-filled cavities, and retinal layers before reaching the photoreceptors in the posterior (back) retina (figure). One of the transparent retinal layers that light passes through is the ganglion cell layer. The ciliary body is a circular structure behind the iris, through which no light passes. The retinal pigment epithelium and choroid are posterior (outer) to the photoreceptors. (Newmark 2006, 21)

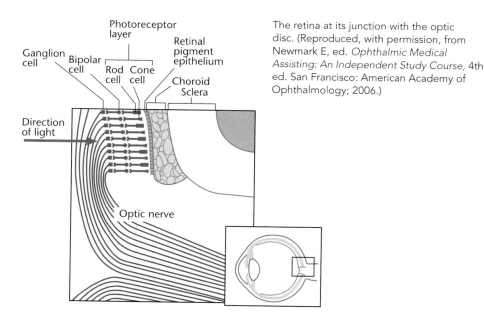

The retina at its junction with the optic disc. (Reproduced, with permission, from Newmark E, ed. *Ophthalmic Medical Assisting: An Independent Study Course*, 4th ed. San Francisco: American Academy of Ophthalmology; 2006.)

10   Melanoma of the choroid is an example of what type of disease?

    a. infectious process
    b. degenerative process
    c. metabolic process
    d. neoplastic process

ANSWER   **d.** neoplastic process

EXPLANATION   A *neoplasm* refers to a solid tissue growth or tumor that may be benign or malignant. Melanoma of the choroid is a malignant tumor ("cancer") that can grow and destroy ocular tissue and spread to other parts of the body (metastasize) and may cause the death of the patient. An infectious process describes a disease caused by bacteria, viruses, fungi, or other microorganisms. *Degeneration* is a term to describe a break down of structure and function mostly due to age, genetics, or other diseases. Metabolic diseases occur from abnormal function of systems elsewhere in the body as seen in diabetes and hypertension. (Newmark 2006, 29–30)

11   Multiple sclerosis (MS) is a chronic disease of the nervous system. It is often associated with what condition?

    a. exophthalmos
    b. scleritis
    c. intermittent droopy eyelids (ptosis)
    d. optic neuritis

ANSWER   **d.** optic neuritis

EXPLANATION   Optic neuritis is inflammation of the optic nerve and is frequently linked with MS. Optic neuritis results in decreased vision, an afferent pupillary defect (APD), and visual field defects. Because the disease is associated with white matter changes of the brain, a magnetic resonance image (MRI) of the brain is typically obtained to confirm the diagnosis of MS. Exophthalmos is common in thyroid disease. Scleritis may be associated with rheumatoid arthritis and other autoimmune conditions. Intermittent ptosis may be due to myasthenia gravis. (Newmark 2006, 46)

12   Exophthalmos often occurs in which disease?

    a. rheumatoid arthritis
    b. Graves disease
    c. diabetes
    d. sarcoidosis

ANSWER   **b.** Graves disease

EXPLANATION   Exophthalmos or proptosis (bulging forward eyeballs) is most commonly caused by Graves disease (hyperthyroidism). (Newmark 2006, 30)

13   What is the correct *general* term when the eyes are not able to fixate on the same visual target due to a misalignment of the globes?

    a. diplopia
    b. exotropia
    c. strabismus
    d. amblyopia

ANSWER   **c.** strabismus

EXPLANATION   Diplopia means *double vision*, which can result from strabismus but is a symptom, not a condition. Exotropia is one form of strabismus, but there are several others. Amblyopia is a loss of vision from disuse of an eye during childhood and is commonly caused by strabismus, but there are other causes. Strabismus is the correct general term for misalignment of the eyes that prevents each eye to fixate on the same visual target. (Newmark 2006, 31)

14   Trichiasis is usually caused by which of the following disorders?

    a. entropion
    b. lagophthalmos
    c. blepharitis
    d. ptosis

ANSWER   **a.** entropion

EXPLANATION   Trichiasis (eyelashes rubbing on the ocular surface) is usually caused by entropion (inturning of the eyelid margin). Lagophthalmos is an inability to fully close the eyelids, blepharitis is an inflammation of the eyelid margin, and ptosis is a droopy eyelid. (Newmark 2006, 33)

15   Ophthalmia neonatorum refers to which condition in a newborn?

    a. conjunctivitis
    b. keratitis
    c. iritis
    d. retinopathy

ANSWER   **a.** conjunctivitis

EXPLANATION   Ophthalmia neonatorum is conjunctivitis in a newborn. Keratitis is an inflammatory process affecting the cornea. Iritis is an inflammatory process affecting the anterior uvea (iris and ciliary body). Retinopathy is a pathologic process involving the retina. (Newmark 2006, 34)

16   A pinguecula is a degeneration of which ocular tissue?

    a. uvea
    b. sclera
    c. cornea
    d. conjunctiva

ANSWER   **d.** conjunctiva

EXPLANATION   A pinguecula is a degeneration of the conjunctiva, forming a small yellowish mass on the temporal or nasal side near the cornea. (Newmark 2006, 35)

17   There are how many extraocular muscles?

    a. 4
    b. 5
    c. 6
    d. 7

ANSWER   **c.** 6

EXPLANATION   There are 6 extraocular muscles: superior rectus, inferior rectus, medial rectus, lateral rectus, superior oblique, and inferior oblique. (Newmark 2006, 13)

18   What is the term for a layer of pus in the anterior chamber?

    a. rubeosis
    b. episcleritis
    c. hypopyon
    d. hyphema

ANSWER   **c.** hypopyon

EXPLANATION   Hypopyon is a layer of white blood cells in the anterior chamber. Rubeosis is the growth of new blood vessels on the iris; episcleritis is an inflammation of the episclera (a tissue layer above the sclera); and hyphema is a layer of red blood cells or blood clot in the anterior chamber. (Newmark 2006, 35)

19   The levator muscle attaches to what structure?

a. tarsus
b. orbicularis
c. conjunctiva
d. sclera

ANSWER   a. tarsus

EXPLANATION   The levator palpebrae muscle, which elevates the upper eyelid, inserts into the tarsus (tarsal plate). The orbicularis muscle closes the eyelids, whereas the conjunctiva and sclera are the outer clear and white layers of the eye, respectively. (Newmark 2006, 15)

20   In primary angle-closure glaucoma, the aqueous outflow channel in the anterior chamber is blocked by which of the following?

a. ciliary body
b. cornea
c. iris
d. lens

ANSWER   c. iris

EXPLANATION   In angle-closure glaucoma, the peripheral iris bows anteriorly and obstructs the aqueous outflow channel causing increased intraocular pressure. (Newmark 2006, 37)

21   Which statement is correct regarding open-angle glaucoma?

a. It is more common earlier in life.
b. It is more common in hyperopia.
c. It is more common in the elderly.
d. It is uninfluenced by corneal thickness.

ANSWER   c. It is more common in the elderly.

EXPLANATION   The risk of developing open-angle glaucoma increases with age. Open-angle glaucoma, sometimes called chronic glaucoma, is more common after age 45. Angle-closure glaucoma is associated with hyperopia. Corneal thickness measurement is an important part of the work-up of a glaucoma patient because there is a relationship between corneal thickness and progression of glaucoma. (Newmark 2006, 37)

22   What does increased intracranial pressure cause?

    a. optic neuritis
    b. ischemic optic neuropathy
    c. glaucoma
    d. papilledema

ANSWER   **d.** papilledema

EXPLANATION   Papilledema is swelling of the optic disc usually in both eyes due to an increase in intracranial pressure; whereas optic neuritis is an inflammation of the optic nerve. Glaucoma is associated with intraocular pressure, and ischemic optic neuropathy is due to occlusion of the blood supply to the optic nerve. (Newmark 2006, 39)

23   What are 2 common ocular manifestations of myasthenia gravis?

    a. ptosis and diplopia
    b. proptosis and dry eye
    c. proptosis and uveitis
    d. ptosis and scleritis

ANSWER   **a.** ptosis and diplopia

EXPLANATION   Ptosis (droopy eyelids) and diplopia (double vision) are 2 common manifestations of myasthenia gravis. Proptosis (bulging forward eyeballs), dry eyes, uveitis (anterior inflammation of the uvea), and scleritis (inflammation of the sclera) are not associated with myasthenia gravis. (Newmark 2006, 44)

24   What disease process is characterized by a reduction in blood flow to an organ or structure?

    a. neoplastic process
    b. metabolic process
    c. infectious process
    d. ischemic process

ANSWER   **d.** ischemic process

EXPLANATION   Ischemic diseases are caused by a lack of blood supply. Examples of ischemic diseases are heart attacks, strokes, and retinal artery occlusions. A neoplastic process is characterized by a growth of tissue, either benign or malignant. Metabolic processes affect the body's ability to convert food sources into energy to drive normal physiology. Infections are diseases caused by microorganisms, including but not limited to bacteria, fungi, viruses, and chlamydiae. (Newmark 2006, 29)

25   A patient with acquired immunity deficiency syndrome (AIDS) is least likely to have an eye infection caused by which of the following?

   a. histoplasmosis
   b. cytomegalovirus
   c. herpes zoster
   d. toxoplasmosis

ANSWER   **a.** histoplasmosis

EXPLANATION   Cytomegalovirus, herpes zoster, and toxoplasmosis are common infections in patients with AIDS. Histoplasmosis occurs in healthy individuals living in endemic areas for this fungal disease (ie, the Mississippi River Valley). (Newmark 2006, 48)

26   A patient suffers from painful skin eruptions across the left side of his forehead that extends onto his left scalp area. What is the most likely condition?

   a. herpes simplex
   b. psoriasis
   c. varicella-zoster
   d. systemic histoplasmosis

ANSWER   **c.** varicella-zoster

EXPLANATION   Varicella-zoster (chickenpox) virus may become active in the form of painful skin eruptions (shingles) that typically appear in an obvious area on 1 side of the body. When the virus affects the forehead, the same-side eye may also become involved (figure). Skin lesions from herpes simplex tend to be less widespread and are usually less painful. Psoriasis presents as thickened, circumscribed areas of scaling skin that may be found on the scalp but rarely on the face. Histoplasmosis is a fungal condition that does not affect the skin but may cause chorioretinal lesions. (Newmark 2006, 49)

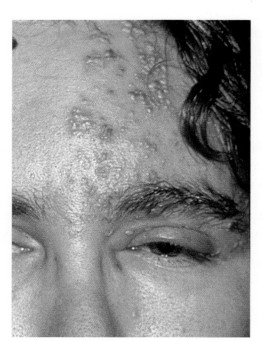

Herpes zoster ophthalmicus. Skin eruptions near the eye and swollen lids. (Reproduced, with permission, from Newmark E, ed. *Ophthalmic Medical Assisting: An Independent Study Course,* 4th ed. San Francisco: American Academy of Ophthalmology; 2006.)

27   What is the range of the wavelengths of visible light?

    a.   80 to 240 centimeters
    b.   400 to 750 nanometers
    c.   4 to 14 kilometers
    d.   360 to 490 millimeters

ANSWER   **b.**   400 to 750 nanometers

EXPLANATION   Light is a form of electromagnetic radiation. What is commonly referred to as light is the very small visible portion of a wide spectrum of electromagnetic radiation (figure). Other forms include cosmic rays, gamma rays, x-rays, ultraviolet rays, infrared rays, and radio waves. The lengths of these electromagnetic rays range from trillionths of a meter to thousands of meters. Visible light occupies only a small area in the center of this spectrum, and the wavelengths of light are expressed in nanometers. The visible light range is 400 to 750 nanometers, or a billionth of a meter. (Newmark 2006, 54)

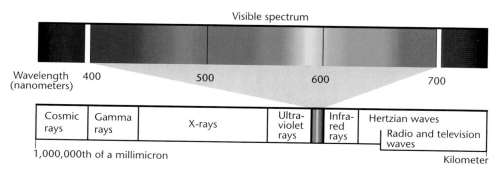

The spectrum of electromagnetic radiation. Note the narrow band of visible light. (Reproduced, with permission, from Newmark E, ed. *Ophthalmic Medical Assisting: An Independent Study Course,* 4th ed. San Francisco: American Academy of Ophthalmology; 2006.)

28   The surface of the normal eye is hydrophobic. What does this term mean?

    a.   It is acidic.
    b.   It is basic.
    c.   It resists water.
    d.   It is water friendly.

ANSWER   **c.**   It resists water.

EXPLANATION   Hydrophobic means *water fearing* or *resists water.* Hydrophobic agents can be acidic or basic. Hydrophilic substances have an affinity for water. Mucin formed by the conjunctival goblet cells allows the tears to wet the ocular surface. (Newmark 2006, 80)

29   An exophthalmometer is used in screening for which of the following?

    a.   glaucoma
    b.   proptosis
    c.   strabismus
    d.   amblyopia

ANSWER   **b.** proptosis

EXPLANATION   The exophthalmometer is an instrument that measures the amount of forward protrusion of the eye beyond the orbital rim (proptosis). Glaucoma is an optic neuropathy related to intraocular pressure. Strabismus is a misalignment of the eyes. Amblyopia refers to decreased vision without apparent abnormality in the eye ("lazy eye") due to visual deprivation during infancy and early childhood. (Newmark 2006, 137)

30   Which of the following patients would be best seen the same day that they call?

    a. a patient previously diagnosed with cataract, with slowly progressive painless loss of vision in 1 eye over the prior 2 to 3 years
    b. a patient with red and itchy eyes for the past month
    c. a patient with sudden and total loss of vision in one eye ½ hour prior to calling
    d. a patient with red eyes and drainage for the previous 2 to 3 days.

ANSWER   **c.** a patient with sudden and total loss of vision in one eye ½ hour prior to calling

EXPLANATION   The patient previously diagnosed with cataract has symptoms most consistent with cataract. While surgery may be needed, this patient does not need to be seen urgently. Red, itchy eyes for a month is neither a serious nor an acute complaint. The patient with red eyes and drainage likely has conjunctivitis, which is usually not a serious condition. Although the patient needs to be seen, an appointment within 24 to 36 hours would be reasonable. Sudden and total loss of vision reflects the acute onset of a serious problem that needs to be seen emergently. A general guideline is that patients should be seen in the same amount of time that they have had symptoms. (Newmark 2006, 215–217)

31   What is the material of choice for safety lenses?

    a. chemically hardened glass
    b. CR39 plastic
    c. polycarbonate plastic
    d. polyurethane plastic

ANSWER   **c.** polycarbonate plastic

EXPLANATION   Polycarbonate lenses are favored for safety glasses because they are light weight, shatter-resistant, and inexpensive. Chemically hardened glass also makes a very good safety lens and it is very scratch resistant. However, it is not commonly used because the lenses are heavier and more expensive than polycarbonate. CR39 plastic and polyurethane lenses shatter much more easily than polycarbonate and chemically hardened glass. (Newmark 2006, 179)

32   Which statement is correct regarding visually impaired patients?

    a. Verbal communication may be more extensive than with normally sighted patients.
    b. Visually impaired patients will not benefit from a low-vision referral.
    c. History-taking is the same as for normally sighted patients.
    d. Visually impaired patients must be accompanied by a friend or family member.

ANSWER   **a.** Verbal communication may be more extensive than with normally sighted patients.

EXPLANATION   Visual impairment can be defined as low vision that cannot be corrected; consequently, verbal communication may be more useful than for patients with unimpaired vision. Patients with low vision or special needs may benefit from a low-vision specialist. Special questions to elicit a functional history are useful for patients with low vision. A patient with low vision may be examined alone but yet benefit from a third-party assistant. (Newmark 2006, 230–231)

33   Which of the following ophthalmic symptoms is most typical for a patient with new-onset diabetes mellitus?

    a. flashing lights and floaters
    b. intermittent droopy eyelids (ptosis)
    c. blurred vision
    d. dry eyes and dry mouth

ANSWER   **c.** blurred vision

EXPLANATION   Fluctuating blood sugar levels may cause changes in the crystalline lens, resulting in a temporary refractive shift and blurred vision. Flashing lights and floaters are typical for a posterior vitreous detachment (PVD). Intermittent ptosis may be indicative of myasthenia gravis. Dry eyes and dry mouth may be associated with Sjögren syndrome. (Newmark 2006, 238)

34   Which of the following applies to a rigid protective eye shield?

    a. protects a lacerated globe
    b. prevents further bleeding
    c. can be glued into place
    d. prevents eyelid movement

ANSWER   **a.** protects a lacerated globe

EXPLANATION   A rigid eye shield protects a recently operated upon eye, eye lacerations, or a perforated globe. An eye shield is taped in place. It does not prevent eyelid movement or bleeding. (Newmark 2006, 254)

35   A diabetic patient starts to have an acute hypoglycemic reaction in the office. What should the ophthalmic technician prepare to do besides notify the doctor?

    a. Check the pupils for symmetry.
    b. Give the patient a quick-acting sugary food.
    c. Call 911.
    d. Give the patient an antiemetic agent.

ANSWER   **b.** Give the patient a quick-acting sugary food.

EXPLANATION   Hypoglycemia results from low blood sugar levels and may result in seizure or coma. Fruit juice or candy may quickly reverse this reaction, eliminating the need to call 911. Vomiting (emesis) is typically not associated with hypoglycemic reactions. Checking the patient's pupils is not helpful. (Newmark 2006, 238)

36   Which part of the eye is involved in focusing light?

   a. cornea
   b. aqueous humor
   c. vitreous
   d. retina

ANSWER   **a.** cornea

EXPLANATION   The cornea and the lens focus light on to the retina. The aqueous humor (the clear fluid between the cornea and lens) and the vitreous (the jelly-like substance between the lens and retina) do not contribute to the focusing power of the eye. (Newmark 2006, 17)

37   In which location do the optic nerve fibers cross?

   a. optic chiasm
   b. optic tracts
   c. lateral geniculate body
   d. visual cortex

ANSWER   **a.** optic chiasm

EXPLANATION   Nerve fibers traveling in the optic nerves of each eye cross in the optic chiasm in the brain. The optic tracts carry the fibers from the chiasm to the lateral geniculate bodies, where they synapse, and then the optic radiations carry the new fibers to the visual cortex. (Newmark 2006, 21–22)

38   If a patient asks you a question about a test result or diagnosis, what is the best action to take?

   a. Give the information to the patient.
   b. Refer the patient to the Internet.
   c. Refer the patient to the ophthalmologist.
   d. Tell the patient you don't know the answer to the question.

ANSWER   **c.** Refer the patient to the ophthalmologist.

EXPLANATION   Even if the medical assistant knows the answer to the patient's question, it is best to refer the patient to the ophthalmologist. Telling the patient that you don't know the answer may not be the truth. The Internet has a great deal of health information, but much of it is not accurate, helpful, or complete. Referring to specific Internet sites that have been reviewed for accuracy may be helpful, but this does not address the patient's immediate query. (Newmark 2006, 117)

39   All **except** which of the following are important in assessing a patient with glaucoma?

    a. measurement of intraocular pressure

    b. measurement of corneal thickness

    c. analysis of aqueous humor from the anterior chamber

    d. visual field examination

ANSWER   **c.** analysis of aqueous humor from the anterior chamber

EXPLANATION   Glaucoma is a disease in which the intraocular pressure is usually elevated that leads to optic nerve damage, manifested by a loss of visual field. Thus, measurement of intraocular pressure and visual field is important in assessing glaucoma. Corneal thickness, measured by a technique called *pachymetry*, has been found to be an important risk factor for glaucoma; hence, its measurement is also important. Analysis of aqueous fluid can be important in the diagnosis of some infectious diseases of the eye, but has no role in the diagnosis and management of glaucoma. (Newmark 2006, 37)

40   All **except** which of the following circumstances might require a pressure patch?

    a. a full-thickness corneal laceration

    b. a corneal abrasion

    c. a recently operated eye that has received a peribulbar anesthetic block

    d. a patient with an exposed eye from 7th cranial nerve palsy

ANSWER   **a.** a full-thickness corneal laceration

EXPLANATION   In an "open globe," with a full-thickness laceration in the wall of the eye, of which the cornea is a part, undue pressure on the eye can worsen the injury by squeezing ocular tissues, such as the iris, lens, or vitreous, out of the eye. Lacerated globes should be covered with a protective shield, but not a pressure patch. Healing of large corneal abrasions is facilitated by pressure patching, which immobilizes the eyelids and prevents the abrasive effect of the lids blinking over the abrasion. After an anesthetic block, the eyelids cannot close properly, and the patch therefore helps to protect the eye. Likewise, an eye with a 7th cranial nerve palsy that cannot blink properly also can benefit from protection from a patch. (Newmark 2006, 254)

41   Common causes of conjunctivitis include all **except** which of the following?

    a. bacteria

    b. allergy

    c. exposure to a sunlamp (UV light)

    d. viruses

ANSWER   **c.** exposure to a sunlamp (UV light)

EXPLANATION   Conjunctivitis (figure) is inflammation of the conjunctiva, the tissue that covers the inner eyelid (palpebral conjunctiva) and outer surface of the eye (bulbar conjunctiva). It is most commonly caused by infections with bacteria or viruses, or by allergy.

Chronic exposure to UV light, such as a sun lamp, may lead to growths on the conjunctiva such as pterygia or tumors. Acute exposure to UV light can cause a keratitis and does not cause conjunctivitis. (Newmark 2006, 33–34)

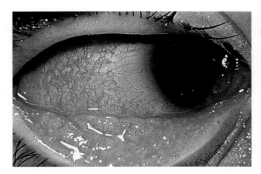

Conjunctival disorders. Conjunctivitis. (Reproduced, with permission, from Newmark E, ed. *Ophthalmic Medical Assisting: An Independent Study Course,* 4th ed. San Francisco: American Academy of Ophthalmology; 2006.)

42 Features of thyroid ophthalmopathy include all **except** which of the following?

a. ptosis
b. proptosis
c. strabismus
d. exposure keratopathy

ANSWER   a. ptosis

EXPLANATION   Features of thyroid eye disease include a forward protrusion of the eye, called *proptosis*, which, along with eyelid retraction, leads to exposure keratopathy (figure). In addition, involvement of the extraocular muscles can lead to a restrictive strabismus. In thyroid eye disease, the eyelids become retracted, or opened too widely, which is the opposite of *ptosis*, which refers to a droopy eyelid. (Newmark 2006, 31, 45–46)

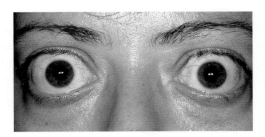

Thyroid ophthalmopathy. Retracted lids and proptosis. (Reproduced, with permission, from Newmark E, ed. *Ophthalmic Medical Assisting: An Independent Study Course,* 4th ed. San Francisco: American Academy of Ophthalmology; 2006.)

43 The retina contains all **except** which of the following cells?

a. goblet cells
b. bipolar cells
c. ganglion cells
d. rod cells

ANSWER   a. goblet cells

EXPLANATION   Goblet cells, which produce mucin, are found in the conjunctiva. All of the other cell types listed are found in the retina. (Newmark 2006, 16)

44   The standard comprehensive eye examination includes all **except** which of the following?

   a. visual acuity
   b. intraocular pressure
   c. exophthalmometry
   d. slit-lamp examination

ANSWER   **c.** exophthalmometry

EXPLANATION   Exophthalmometry is not part of the standard comprehensive eye examination. Exophthalmometry measures the prominence of the eyeballs in relation to the bony orbital rim. The measurement is performed with an instrument called an *exophthalmometer* (figure). It is employed with patients whose eyeballs are bulging, as seen in hyperthyroid disease. Visual acuity, intraocular pressure measurement, and the slit lamp examination (among others) are all part of the standard comprehensive eye examination. (Newmark 2006, 112, 137)

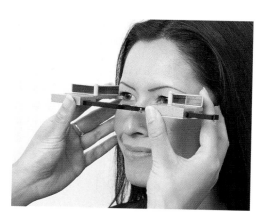

Measurements of proptosis with an exophthalmometer. (Reproduced, with permission, from Wilson FM, ed. *Practical Ophthalmology,* 6th ed. San Francisco: American Academy of Ophthalmology; 2009.)

45   The uveal tract consists of all **except** which of the following?

   a. ciliary body
   b. inner limiting membrane
   c. choroid
   d. iris

ANSWER   **b.** inner limiting membrane

EXPLANATION   The uveal tract is the pigmented, vascular layer of the eye (figure). It exists as a continuous layer formed by the iris anteriorly, ciliary body in the middle, and choroid posterior. The inner limiting membrane is the innermost layer of the retina. (Newmark 2006, 37)

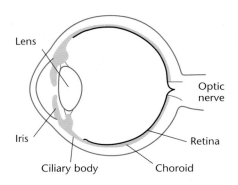

The uveal tract. The iris, ciliary body, and choroid in relation to other structures of the eye. (Reproduced, with permission, from Newmark E, ed. *Ophthalmic Medical Assisting: An Independent Study Course,* 4th ed. San Francisco: American Academy of Ophthalmology; 2006.)

46   What condition does **not** develop during adulthood?

    a. amblyopia

    b. macular degeneration

    c. cataract

    d. glaucoma

ANSWER   **a.** amblyopia

EXPLANATION   Amblyopia (lazy eye) is a condition that develops when vision development is suppressed during childhood. Cataract, macular degeneration, and glaucoma are most commonly diseases of adulthood; although cataract and glaucoma are seen in infancy and early childhood, they are very uncommon. Amblyopia is a condition that develops only in childhood. (Newmark 2006, 14)

47   Which of the following is **not** a manifestation of rheumatoid arthritis?

    a. scleritis

    b. dry eye

    c. peripheral corneal ulceration

    d. follicular conjunctivitis

ANSWER   **d.** follicular conjunctivitis

EXPLANATION   Rheumatoid arthritis is a systemic inflammatory disease that can affect external ocular structures and is a common cause of scleritis and peripheral corneal ulceration (figure). Sjögren syndrome, which is most commonly associated with rheumatoid arthritis, causes a dry eye and dry mouth. Follicular conjunctivitis is usually an infectious disease caused by viruses and chlamydial organisms, and is not a manifestation of rheumatoid arthritis. (Newmark 2006, 44)

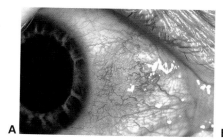 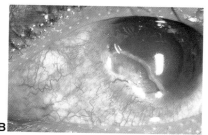

Ocular manifestations of rheumatoid arthritis. (A) Scleritis. (B) Corneal ulcer (Reproduced, with permission, from Newmark E, ed. *Ophthalmic Medical Assisting: An Independent Study Course*, 4th ed. San Francisco: American Academy of Ophthalmology; 2006.)

48   Which of the following is **not** correct regarding keratoconjunctivitis sicca?

    a. A dry mouth may be associated.
    b. Lubricants are often used for treatment.
    c. The lacrimal punctum should be dilated.
    d. The patient may have arthritis.

ANSWER   **c.** The lacrimal punctum should be dilated.

EXPLANATION   Dilating the lacrimal punctum would worsen the symptoms of dry eye in a patient with keratoconjunctivitis sicca. Closing the punctum with silicone plugs is a possible treatment of keratoconjunctivitis sicca. A dry mouth is often associated with this condition, as is arthritis. Lubricants are often used for treatment. (Newmark 2006, 44–45)

49   Which of the following is **not** found in the anterior segment of the eye?

    a. aqueous humor
    b. choroid
    c. Schlemm's canal
    d. lens

ANSWER   **b.** choroid

EXPLANATION   The choroid is the vascular layer that provides nutrition for the retina, and is therefore part of the posterior segment of the eye. The anterior segment of the eye is everything anterior to the vitreous. This would include the cornea; the anterior and posterior chambers, which contain the aqueous humor; the iris; the ciliary body; and the lens. Schlemm's canal is located in the anterior chamber angle, which is formed by the junction of the iris and cornea, so it is in the anterior segment. (Newmark 2006, 17–20).

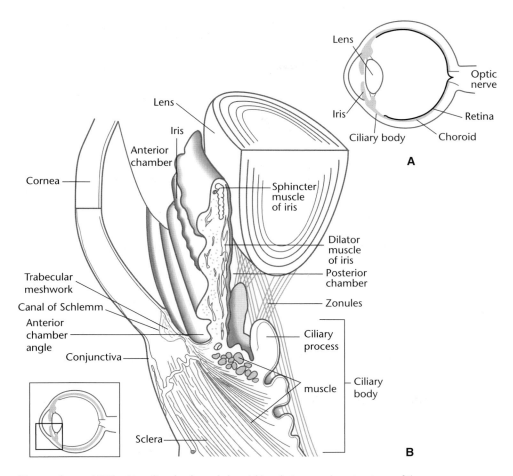

The uveal tract. (A) The iris, ciliary body, and choroid in relation to other structures of the eye. (B) Details of the uveal structure. (Reproduced, with permission, from Newmark E, ed. *Ophthalmic Medical Assisting: An Independent Study Course,* 4th ed. San Francisco: American Academy of Ophthalmology; 2006.)

50 Which of the following is **not** part of the cardiovascular system?

a. ophthalmic artery
b. central retinal vein
c. aqueous vein
d. carotid artery

ANSWER c. aqueous vein

EXPLANATION The cardiovascular system includes the heart, which pumps blood throughout the body; the arteries, which carry blood to organs and tissues; capillaries; and veins, which carry blood back to the heart. The carotid artery supplies blood to the brain and eye; the ophthalmic artery supplies blood to the eye and orbit; and the central retinal vein drains blood from the eye. These are all part of the cardiovascular system. The aqueous vein (figure) drains aqueous humor, not blood, from the eye, and it therefore is not part of the cardiovascular system. (Newmark 2006, 44; Trobe 2006, 111)

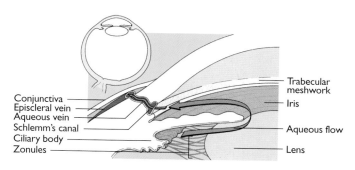

Primary open-angle glaucoma. Normal flow of aqueous. (Reproduced, with permission, from Trobe JD, *The Physician's Guide to Eye Care,* 3rd ed. San Francisco: American Academy of Ophthalmology; 2006.)

51   Which of the following is **not** part of the ophthalmic medical assistant's responsibilities?

    a. Estimate visual acuity.
    b. Measure intraocular pressure.
    c. Diagnose a condition.
    d. Take a history.

ANSWER   **c.** Diagnose a condition.

EXPLANATION   An ophthalmic medical assistant can assist the physician with the visual acuity testing, intraocular pressure measurement, and history-taking. However, the assistant should not interpret tests, diagnose a condition, or treat a patient's condition without the doctor's express instructions. (Newmark 2006, 6)

52   Which of the following is **not** part of the triage process?

    a. determining the nature of the patient's complaint
    b. determining the severity of the patient's complaint
    c. determining the duration of the patient's complaint
    d. a medical review of systems

ANSWER   **d.** a medical review of systems

EXPLANATION   Triage is the process by which one evaluates a patient's problem and the urgency with which that patient should be seen. Some problems are more urgent than others: pain or loss of vision is more urgent than itching of the eye. The more severe the problem is, the more urgent the triage level is. For example, a patient complaining of complete loss of vision is more urgent to see than a patient with a little blurring. In addition, a good general rule is that the shorter the duration of the complaint, the sooner a patient should be seen. While the review of systems is an important part of the medical history, it is not relevant in the determination of the urgency of the problem. (Newmark 2006, 214–217)

53   Which of the following steps does **not** apply to the process of applying a pressure patch to the eye?

    a. The eye is anesthetized.
    b. A folded patch is used.
    c. Tape is placed on the forehead.
    d. The cheek is pulled up toward the forehead.

ANSWER   **a.** The eye is anesthetized.

EXPLANATION   The eye does not need to be anesthetized to get pressure patched. First, the forehead and the area around the cheekbone and toward the ear are cleaned with an alcohol pad to remove skin oils. Two sterile pads are used; the one closest to the eye is folded over. The patient is asked to close both eyes tightly. The unfolded pad is taped firmly to the forehead with a 5- to 6-inch length of adhesive surgical tape, and brought down, toward the cheekbone. The cheek is pulled up toward the forehead prior to affixing the lower end of the tape. This makes the patch tight against the eye to prevent the eyelids from opening under the patch. (Newmark 2006, 254)

54   Which of the following structures is **not** found in the normal eyelid?

    a. bulbar conjunctiva
    b. orbicularis oculi muscle
    c. cilia
    d. meibomian glands

ANSWER   **a.** bulbar conjunctiva

EXPLANATION   The palpebral conjunctiva forms the inner layer of the eyelid; the bulbar conjunctiva covers the sclera, and therefore is not part of the eyelid. The orbicularis muscle is the muscle that closes the eyelids. *Cilia* is a term for eyelashes, which are obviously found in the eyelid. The meibomian glands are oil-secreting glands, which are found in the tarsal plate, a structure that gives the eyelids their firmness and shape. The figures show the external eyelids and a cross section. (Newmark 2006, 14–15)

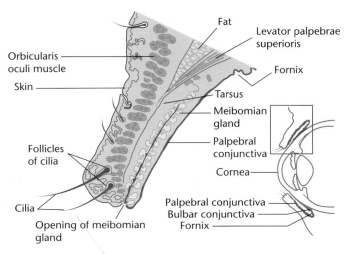

The external eyelids. (Reproduced, with permission, from Newmark E, ed. *Ophthalmic Medical Assisting: An Independent Study Course,* 4th ed. San Francisco: American Academy of Ophthalmology; 2006.)

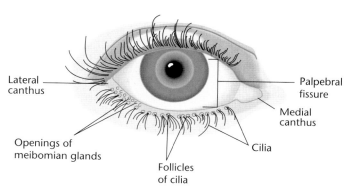

Cross section of the eyelid. (Reproduced, with permission, from Newmark E, ed. *Ophthalmic Medical Assisting: An Independent Study Course,* 4th ed. San Francisco: American Academy of Ophthalmology; 2006.)

55   Which of the following structures is **not** involved in creating a focused visual image?

   a. lens
   b. cornea
   c. vitreous
   d. retina

ANSWER   **c.** vitreous

EXPLANATION   The vitreous (figure), under normal conditions, is optically clear and does not contribute to image formation. The cornea and lens are structures whose purpose is to focus a clear image on the retina. The distance of the retina from the cornea and lens determines whether a clear image can be formed, and the retina then transmits that image to the visual cortex. (Newmark 2006, 12)

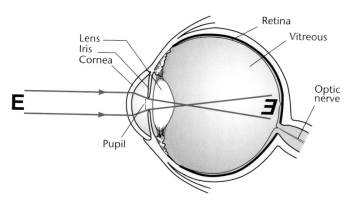

The eye as an optical system. (Reproduced, with permission, from Newmark E, ed. *Ophthalmic Medical Assisting: An Independent Study Course,* 4th ed. San Francisco: American Academy of Ophthalmology; 2006.)

56   Which of the following structures is **not** involved in the drainage of tears?

   a. canaliculus
   b. punctum
   c. nasolacrimal duct
   d. accessory lacrimal gland

ANSWER   **d.** accessory lacrimal gland

EXPLANATION   The figure shows the lacrimal apparatus. Draining tears enter an opening in the medial aspect of the eyelid, called the *punctum*, pass through a tubular structure called a *canaliculus*, enter the lacrimal sac, and then drain into the nose through the nasolacrimal duct. Accessory lacrimal glands are involved in the production, not the drainage, of tears. (Newmark 2006, 16)

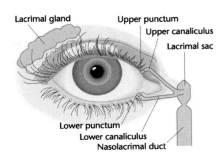

The lacrimal apparatus. (Reproduced, with permission, from Newmark E, ed. *Ophthalmic Medical Assisting: An Independent Study Course,* 4th ed. San Francisco: American Academy of Ophthalmology; 2006.)

57   Which of the following substances is **not** a hormone produced by the endocrine system?

   a. insulin
   b. cholesterol
   c. estrogen
   d. thyroxine

ANSWER   **b.** cholesterol

EXPLANATION   The endocrine system includes several glands that produce hormones, which are substances that regulate physiologic processes. These include insulin, which controls sugar metabolism; estrogen, which regulates female sexual development and function; and thyroxine, a thyroid hormone, which regulates metabolic processes. Cholesterol is a product of lipid metabolism that does not have any regulatory function. (Newmark 2006, 44)

58   Which statement is **incorrect** concerning herpes simplex virus?

   a. It causes a corneal infection characterized by a dendritic pattern.
   b. It causes fever blisters or "cold sores."
   c. Corneal infection can lead to scarring.
   d. It causes shingles.

ANSWER   **d.** It causes shingles.

EXPLANATION   Herpes simplex is a common cause of eye infections, the most common of which is a corneal infection (keratitis) characterized by a dendritic pattern on corneal staining with fluorescein. It is the same virus that causes fever blisters, and the keratitis can be considered a fever blister on the eye. Prolonged infection can lead to corneal scarring, and this is a common reason for corneal transplantation. Shingles is not caused by herpes simplex, but by a closely related virus called the varicella-zoster virus. (Newmark 2006, 49)

59   Which statement is **incorrect** regarding diabetes mellitus?

  a. Diabetes can affect peripheral nerves, kidneys, and eyes.
  b. Diabetes is a common cause of blindness.
  c. Diabetic retinopathy risk is not altered by a higher blood pressure and hemoglobin A_{1C} level.
  d. Laser treatment is an effective treatment for diabetic retinopathy.

ANSWER   **c.** Diabetic retinopathy risk is not altered by a higher blood pressure and hemoglobin A_{1C} level.

EXPLANATION   Diabetes is a common cause of peripheral neuropathy, renal failure, and retinopathy. It is a leading cause of blindness with a 25× greater risk of blindness compared to people without diabetes. Laser treatment can be effective for both proliferative and nonproliferative retinopathy. The risk of retinopathy is reduced by blood pressures less than 140/85 and hemoglobin A_{1C} levels less than 7%. (Newmark 2006, 46–47)

60   Which statement is **incorrect** regarding HIV infection and AIDS?

  a. Human immunodeficiency virus (HIV) can be transmitted only by sexual contact.
  b. Cytomegalovirus (CMV) retinitis is a common ocular manifestation of acquired immunodeficiency syndrome (AIDS).
  c. Antiretroviral drugs prolong the life of AIDS patients.
  d. AIDS-related infections occur most commonly in patients with CD4 lymphocyte counts less than 50.

ANSWER   **a.** Human immunodeficiency virus (HIV) can be transmitted only by sexual contact.

EXPLANATION   AIDS patients can develop a variety of ocular infections that necessitate visits to the ophthalmologist. CMV retinitis is the most common of these and is associated with low CD4 lymphocyte counts. Current treatment with highly active antiretroviral treatment (HAART) protocols has greatly increased the life expectancy of HIV-infected patients. HIV is most commonly transmitted by sexual contact, but can also be transmitted by any exchange of bodily fluids, especially blood transfusions. It is also potentially possible (but has never been documented) to transmit the virus through ocular fluids, so it is important to have protocols to properly sterilize ocular exam equipment, such as tonometer tips, that come in contact with AIDS patients. (Newmark 2006, 48)

61   Which of the following is **not** an ocular manifestation of a systemic disease?

  a. glaucoma
  b. diabetic retinopathy
  c. Sjögren syndrome
  d. proptosis with exposure keratopathy

ANSWER   **a.** glaucoma

EXPLANATION   Systemic diseases are those that have effects throughout the body. Diabetes affects sugar metabolism and blood vessels throughout the body, including the eye. Sjögren syndrome is an autoimmune disease associated with other autoimmune diseases such as rheumatoid arthritis and systemic lupus erythematosus (SLE), and can cause a dry eye. Proptosis with exposure keratopathy is most commonly caused by Graves disease, an endocrine disease that affects the thyroid gland and metabolism throughout the body. Glaucoma is a disease that is limited to the eye. (Newmark 2006, 44–47)

12 OPHTHALMIC IMAGING

1   Which of the following images depicts the fundus camera?

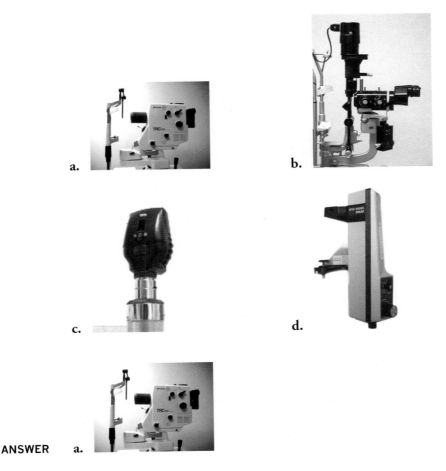

a.

b.

c.

d.

ANSWER   a.

EXPLANATION   The image in "a" is a typical fundus camera setup that can also be used for intravenous fundus fluorescein or indocyanine green (ICG) angiography. The image in "b" represents a slit-lamp biomicroscope. The image in "c" is a direct ophthalmoscope. The image in "d" is a potential acuity meter (PAM). (Newmark 2006, 146)

(Images reproduced, with permission, from Miller KM, *Basic and Clinical Science Course,* Section 3: Clinical Optics, American Academy of Ophthalmology, 2006–2007. All parts courtesy of Neal H. Atebara, MD.)

2   The most accurate method of performing a B-scan ultrasound is through what approach?

    a. with the probe and ultrasound gel in direct contact on the closed eyelid

    b. with the probe held over the area of interest, but not in direct contact with the patient

    c. with the probe and ultrasound gel in direct contact on the surface of the anesthetized eye

    d. with the probe without ultrasound gel in direct contact on the surface of the anesthetized eye

ANSWER   **c.** with the probe and ultrasound gel in direct contact on the surface of the anesthetized eye

EXPLANATION   While it is possible to perform B-scan ultrasound through the closed eyelid with ultrasound gel, the most accurate results for a B-scan ultrasound are obtained with the use of the probe and ultrasound gel being in direct contact with the anesthetized eye (figure). (Newmark 2006, 148; Waldron 1999, 1–14)

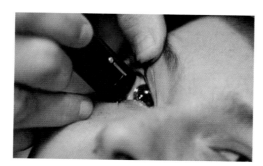

Proper probe position on the globe, with the patient looking in the direction of the pathology, and the probe opposite with the marker oriented superiorly. (Image by Jorge Rodriguez, courtesy of Denice Barsness, CRA, COMT, ROUB, FOPS.)

3   What is the best photographic test to document the size, appearance, and location of an atypical choroidal nevus?

    a. fundus photography

    b. external photography

    c. slit-lamp photography

    d. specular microscopy photography

ANSWER   **a.** fundus photography

EXPLANATION   The appearance, size, and location of choroidal nevi (freckles) can often be adequately documented with posterior segment imaging tests like fundus photography (figure). The ophthalmologist may also order fundus fluorescein angiography to further characterize the fundus lesion. External photography images the eye's outer structures. Slit-lamp photography images the anterior structures of the globe. Specular microscopy photography images the corneal endothelium. (Newmark 2006, 145)

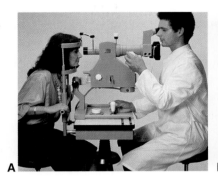
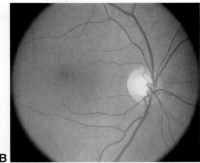

(A) Fundus photography of the retina. (B) Resulting photograph showing normal retina. (Reproduced, with permission, from Newmark E, ed. *Ophthalmic Medical Assisting: An Independent Study Course,* 4th ed. San Francisco: American Academy of Ophthalmology; 2006.)

4   What is the function of angling the slit beam in slit-lamp photography?

a. serves as the gold-standard for measuring corneal thickness
b. allows one to see deeper into the eye
c. provides visualization of the limbus
d. provides an appreciation of depth

ANSWER   d. provides an appreciation of depth

EXPLANATION   As in the ordinary slit-lamp examination, the angled slit-beam in slit-lamp photography provides an appreciation of relative depth. An optical system that uses the slit beam to measure the corneal thickness does not require angulation. Angulation is not required to view the limbus or penetrate deep into the eye. (Newmark 2006, 145)

5   What is the function of the corneal endothelial cells?

a. prevents the entrance of bacteria, viruses, and fungi into the eye
b. acts as a pump to keep fluid out of the corneal layers to keep it clear
c. maintains elasticity of the cornea to protect it from damage
d. produces fluid to the keep the anterior chamber formed

ANSWER   b. acts as a pump to keep fluid out of the corneal layers to keep it clear

EXPLANATION   The corneal endothelial cells function as a pump to keep fluid out of the corneal layers. If there are not enough endothelial cells, due to trauma or a condition known as Fuchs corneal dystrophy, the cornea may fill with fluid and become cloudy. Specular microscopy is used to evaluate the corneal endothelial cells (figure). (Newmark 2006, 145)

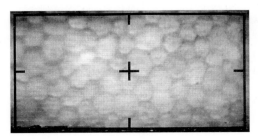

Specular photograph showing normal endothelial cells. (Reproduced, with permission, from Newmark E, *Ophthalmic Medical Assisting: An Independent Study Course,* 4th ed. San Francisco: American Academy of Ophthalmology; 2006.)

6   What test uses concentric lighted rings (Placido disks) to visually and quantitatively depict the amount of astigmatism present in the cornea?

    a. corneal topography
    b. specular microscopy
    c. slit-lamp photography
    d. scanning laser polarimetry (GDx)

ANSWER   **a.** corneal topography

EXPLANATION   The distortions of the reflected rings used with corneal topography are analyzed to produce a detailed map of the corneal curvature (power), showing steeper and flatter areas and irregularities. Specular microscopy images the corneal endothelium. Slit-lamp photography images the anterior ocular structures. Scanning laser polarimetry (GDx) measures the retinal nerve fiber layer thickness surrounding the optic disc. (Newmark 2006, 145)

7   What type of photography requires a close-up lens with an electronic flash attachment?

    a. fundus photography
    b. external photography
    c. corneal topography
    d. scanning laser polarimetry

ANSWER   **b.** external photography

EXPLANATION   To obtain adequate images of the eye's outer structures (eg, an eyelid tumor), a still camera equipped with a close-up "macro" lens and an electronic flash attachment is all that is required. (Newmark 2006, 145)

8   A fundus fluorescein angiogram typically highlights details of the retinal vasculature. Fundus indocyanine green (ICG) angiography typically highlights details of what vascular system?

    a. iris vasculature
    b. choroidal vasculature
    c. optic nerve vasculature
    d. ciliary body vasculature

ANSWER   **b.** choroidal vasculature

EXPLANATION   ICG angiography utilizes ICG dye that is able to penetrate more deeply into the eye behind the retina to highlight details of the choroidal blood vessels. Although the iris blood vessels can be imaged with ICG dye, this is an atypical use of this dye. The optic nerve vasculature and ciliary body vasculature cannot be imaged by fundus photography with ICG angiography. (Newmark 2006, 146–147)

9   Patients undergoing intravenous fundus fluorescein angiography frequently report what common side effect?

   a. dizziness
   b. chest pain
   c. tingling in their hands and feet
   d. nausea

ANSWER   **d.** nausea

EXPLANATION   Although more serious side effects of intravenous fundus fluorescein angiography can rarely occur (eg, anaphylactic shock), nausea is a commonly encountered symptom that typically does not require the test to be canceled. (Newmark 2006, 147)

10   Intravenous fundus fluorescein angiography is the test that is most helpful in determining the presence or absence of which of the following?

   a. guttata
   b. retinal or choroidal neovascularization
   c. meibomian gland dysfunction
   d. phlyctenules

ANSWER   **b.** retinal or choroidal neovascularization

EXPLANATION   Guttata (little bumps in the endothelial cell layer) are found on the back surface of the cornea with slit-lamp photography or endothelial microscopy. Meibomian gland dysfunction and corneal phlyctenules (blisters) can be documented with slit-lamp photography. Neovascularization is the abnormal growth of new blood vessels. Leakage of dye from neovascularization of the retina (eg, in patients with proliferative diabetic retinopathy) or the choroid (eg, in patients with neovascular age-related macular degeneration) is best observed with intravenous fundus fluorescein angiography (figure). (Newmark 2006, 146–147)

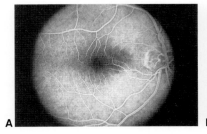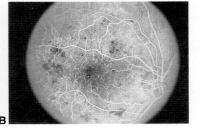

Retinal angiography. (A) Fluorescein angiogram of a normal retina. (B) Fluorescein angiogram of a diabetic patient. The numerous white dots are tiny outpouchings in abnormal capillaries (microaneurysms) that are filling up with dye. (Reproduced, with permission, from Newmark E, ed. *Ophthalmic Medical Assisting: An Independent Study Course,* 4th ed. San Francisco: American Academy of Ophthalmology; 2006.)

11   Pharmacologic dilation of the pupil (mydriasis) is absolutely required for which of the following tests?

    a. fundus photography
    b. optical coherence tomography
    c. external photography
    d. slit-lamp photography

ANSWER   **a.** fundus photography

EXPLANATION   External photography and slit-lamp photography do not absolutely require pharmacologic dilation of the pupil, though it may be helpful for retroillumination with slit-lamp photography in certain circumstances. Optical coherence tomography images are much easier to obtain in the pharmacologically dilated pupil, but mydriasis is not absolutely required in every case. In order to obtain adequate visualization of the optic nerve, macula, and post-equatorial retina with fundus photography, one must have a pharmacologically dilated pupil. (Newmark 2006, 146)

12   Slit-lamp photography is useful for documentation of which of the following?

    a. structure of the anterior chamber of the eye
    b. optic nerve notch
    c. ciliary body cysts
    d. retinal blood vessel abnormalities

ANSWER   **a.** structure of the anterior chamber of the eye

EXPLANATION   Slit-lamp photography is used to document the anterior segment of the eye, which includes the cornea, anterior chamber, iris, angle, and lens. Fundus photography is used to document the optic nerve and retinal blood vessels. A ciliary body cyst cannot be photographed with a slit lamp because the ciliary body is posterior to the iris and obstructs its view. (Newmark 2006, 146)

13   The Heidelberg retinal tomograph (HRT), optical coherence tomography (OCT), and GDx scanning laser polarimeter with variable corneal compensation are all used to measure what finding and assess what condition?

    a. retinal thickness; pseudophakic cystoid macular edema
    b. retinal thickness; age-related macular degeneration
    c. retinal nerve fiber layer thickness; diabetic retinopathy
    d. retinal nerve fiber layer thickness; glaucoma

ANSWER   **d.** retinal nerve fiber layer thickness; glaucoma

EXPLANATION   All of the imaging tests listed can be used to assess the thickness of the retinal nerve fiber layer in the peripapillary region, the area near or around the optic disc. This information can be used along with intraocular pressure measurements (tonometry), the appearance of the optic nerve, corneal thickness measurements (pachymetry), and the results of a visual field test (perimetry) to determine the extent glaucoma may be troubling the patient. While the OCT is also the gold standard to assess retinal thickness, cystoid macular edema, and age related macular degeneration, the GDx test is not used for this assessment. (Newmark 2006, 147)

14   What individuals need to be present to perform intravenous fundus fluorescein or indocyanine green (ICG) angiography?

    a. registered nurse only
    b. ophthalmic assistant and photographer
    c. physician with or without a photographer
    d. photographer only

ANSWER   **c.** physician with or without a photographer

EXPLANATION   Because of the risk of anaphylactic shock—especially with intravenous fundus fluorescein angiography—a physician and emergency equipment should be on hand during fundus angiography employing intravenous dyes. (Newmark 2006, 147)

15   What tests are the most helpful in confirming the diagnosis of a full-thickness macular hole?

    a. optical coherence tomography and fundus photography
    b. optical coherence tomography and B-scan (B-mode) ultrasonography
    c. optical coherence tomography and intravenous fundus fluorescein angiography
    d. optical coherence tomography and intravenous indocyanine green angiography

ANSWER   **c.** optical coherence tomography and intravenous fundus fluorescein angiography

EXPLANATION   A full-thickness macular hole is traditionally diagnosed by the clinician using slit-lamp fundus biomicroscopy with hand-held condensing lenses. However, the diagnosis can be confirmed with intravenous fundus fluorescein angiography and optical coherence tomography. (Newmark 2006, 147)

16   Which of the following is fluorescein angiography most helpful at characterizing?

    a. drusen
    b. retinal detachment
    c. myelinated nerve fiber
    d. vascular obstruction of blood vessels

ANSWER   **d.** vascular obstruction of blood vessels

EXPLANATION   Fluorescein angiography makes it possible to view detail in blood vessels of the eye, such as vascular obstructions, leakage, and neovascularization. Drusen, myelinated nerve fibers, and retinal detachments can be documented by color fundus photography. (Newmark 2006, 147)

17   Which of the following relationships is correct?

    a. A-scan ultrasonography and lensometry
    b. A-scan ultrasonography and biometry
    c. specular microscopy and keratometry
    d. specular microscopy and pachymetry

ANSWER   **b.** A-scan ultrasonography and biometry

EXPLANATION   Lensometry is a method of determining the prescription of a spectacle (eyeglass) lens. Keratometry is a method of measuring the power of the cornea. Pachymetry is a method of determining the thickness of the cornea. Specular microscopy determines the shape and number of corneal endothelial cells. Biometry is the use of A-scan ultrasonography (also known as *echography*) to determine the length of the eye for intraocular lens calculations. (Newmark 2006, 147)

18   Which ophthalmic imaging test employs light to create a cross-sectional image of the retina using false coloration?

    a. A-scan (A-mode) biometry
    b. B-scan (B-mode) echography
    c. optical coherence tomography (OCT)
    d. intravenous fundus fluorescein angiography

ANSWER   **c.** optical coherence tomography (OCT)

EXPLANATION   Optical coherence tomography generates a cross-sectional, false-color image of the retina using a laser light source. This allows the ophthalmologist to determine if macular edema, subretinal fluid, or vitreoretinal tractional abnormalities are present in the macula. OCT can also be used to assess the thickness of the retinal nerve fiber layer in the peripapillary area of patients who are being followed for glaucoma. The peripapillary area is the area near or around the optic disc. A-scan and B-scan tests use ultrasound to create images. Intravenous fundus fluorescein angiography is a black-and-white photographic image of the retinal structures. (Newmark 2006, 147)

19   Indocyanine green angiography is used specifically to study what part of the eye?

    a. angle structure of the eye
    b. zonular structure of the eye
    c. iris structure of the eye
    d. choroidal circulation of the eye

ANSWER   **d.** choroidal circulation of the eye

EXPLANATION   Indocyanine green angiography is used specifically to study the choroidal circulation of the eye. The angle structures of the eye are best studied with gonioscopy, a method of viewing the structures through a special contact lens. The iris structure of the eye can be studied with fluorescein angiography, anterior segment photography, and slit-lamp exam. Although not clinically mainstream, ultrasound biomicroscopy can detect some abnormalities of the zonular structures. (Newmark 2006, 146–147)

20   Which of the following tests should **not** be used if a patient has a documented history of shellfish or iodine allergies?

  a. fluorescein angiography
  b. indocyanine green angiography
  c. slit-lamp photography
  d. applanation tonometry

ANSWER   **b.** indocyanine green angiography

EXPLANATION   Indocyanine green dye contains iodine, which can cause an allergic reaction similar to a shellfish allergy. Intravenous fluorescein can commonly cause nausea, but rarely does a severe allergic reaction occur. There are no dyes used in slit-lamp photography. In applanation tonometry, fluorescein dye is used topically and generally has no systemic side effects when used topically. (Newmark 2006, 147)

21   Which of the following is **not** a common side effect of fluorescein angiography?

  a. severe allergic reaction
  b. hives
  c. nausea
  d. yellow coloration of the urine

ANSWER   **a.** severe allergic reaction

EXPLANATION   Fluorescein angiography is performed with the fundus camera after a fluorescent dye has been injected into a vein in the patient's arm. Severe allergic reactions to fluorescein dye are rare and include difficulty breathing. The dye temporarily discolors the urine and skin. Less than 4% of all patients have nausea, headaches, upset stomach, vomiting, fainting, hives, or itching. (Newmark 2006, 147; Niffenegger 2000, 2–3)

22   What types of images are **not** obtained with a fundus camera with angiography capabilities?

  a. 35-mm film color fundus photographs
  b. digital color fundus photographs
  c. 35-mm film color fundus fluorescein angiography images
  d. digital black-and-white fluorescein angiography images

ANSWER   **c.** 35-mm film color fundus fluorescein angiography images

EXPLANATION   A fundus camera with angiography capabilities typically has a 35-mm camera back or a digital camera back. The camera will provide color and red-free images of the fundus; however, for fluorescein angiography, the camera produces only black-and-white images of the fundus. (Newmark 2006, 146)

13 REFRACTOMETRY

1 Patients with hyperopia may see more clearly with what kind of lens?

    a. plus power diverging lens
    b. minus power diverging lens
    c. plus power converging lens
    d. minus power converging lens

ANSWER **c.** plus power converging lens

EXPLANATION All plus power lenses cause light rays to converge; all minus power lenses cause light rays to diverge. In hyperopia (farsightedness), consider the eyeball is shorter than average, so the converging power of the cornea and lens are not enough to bring the focus point of the light onto the retina. A plus power lens is needed for additional convergence of the light rays. The figure shows refractive characteristics of plus and minus lenses. (Newmark 2006, 57–58)

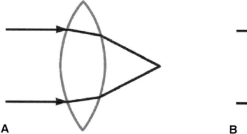 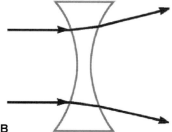

Pair of prisms smoothed to form a convex lens (A) and a concave lens (B), and the subsequent matching refractive characteristics of the lenses. (Reproduced, with permission, from Newmark E, ed. *Ophthalmic Medical Assisting: An Independent Study Course,* 4th ed. San Francisco: American Academy of Ophthalmology; 2006.)

2 In a myopic eye, where are images of distant objects focused?

    a. on the retina
    b. in front of the retina
    c. behind the retina
    d. 1 mm posterior to the crystalline lens

ANSWER **b.** in front of the retina

EXPLANATION Myopia is a condition in which the cornea and lens of the nonaccommodating eye have too much plus power, resulting in images focused in front of the retina. The emmetropic eye focuses distant objects on the retina. The hyperopic eye focuses behind the retina. The figure shows examples of myopia, emmetropia, and hyperopia. (Newmark 2006, 58)

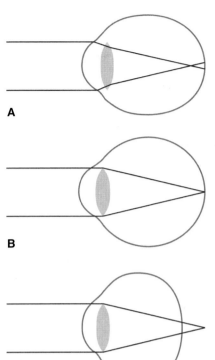

In the myopic eye (A), parallel rays of light are brought to a focus in front of the retina. In the emmetropic eye (B), parallel rays of light focus sharply on the retina. In the hyperopic eye (C), parallel rays of light would come to a focus behind the retina in the unaccommodated eye. (Reproduced, with permission, from Newmark E, ed. *Ophthalmic Medical Assisting: An Independent Study Course,* 4th ed. San Francisco: American Academy of Ophthalmology; 2006.)

3   Why is retinoscopy used?

a. to check for vitreous floaters
b. to inspect the retina
c. to find the fixation point of the eye
d. to objectively estimate the refractive error of the eye

ANSWER   **d.** to objectively estimate the refractive error of the eye

EXPLANATION   Retinoscopy objectively estimates the refractive error by observing how light is reflected back out of the eye. Direct or indirect ophthalmoscopy can be used to inspect the retina and to check for vitreous floaters. A direct ophthalmoscope with a fixation target can be used to find the fixation point of the eye. (Newmark 2006, 64)

4   A cylindrical lens corrects what type of refractive error?

a. myopia
b. hyperopia
c. astigmatism
d. presbyopia

ANSWER   **c.** astigmatism

EXPLANATION   Cylindrical lenses correct astigmatism, spherical lenses correct myopia or hyperopia, and spherocylindrical lenses correct combinations of astigmatism with either myopia or hyperopia. Presbyopia is corrected with additional magnifying power (add) over the distance correction. (Newmark 2006, 61)

5   What is the focal length of a 3.00 D convex lens?

    a. 0.33 m
    b. 0.1 m
    c. 1.0 m
    d. 3.0 m

ANSWER   **a.** 0.33 m

EXPLANATION   A 3.00 D convex lens has a focal length of 1/3 or 0.33 m. The formula to convert diopters into focal length is $D = 1/f$ in meters. (Newmark 2006, 57)

6   Where is the focal point of a hyperopic eye located?

    a. in front of the retina
    b. on the retina
    c. behind the retina
    d. in front of the lens

ANSWER   **c.** behind the retina

EXPLANATION   In a hyperopic eye (farsighted), light is focused behind the retina. Light is focused in front of the retina in a myopic eye (nearsighted) and on the retina in an emmetropic eye (normal or plano). (Newmark 2006, 58)

7   The axis of a cylinder is located how many degrees from its meridian of curvature (power)?

    a. 30°
    b. 60°
    c. 90°
    d. 180°

ANSWER   **c.** 90°

EXPLANATION   The axis and meridian of curvature of a cylinder are separated by 90°. (Newmark 2006, 61)

8   A toric lens is the same as which of the following?

    a. sphere
    b. vertex
    c. spherocylinder
    d. prism

ANSWER   **c.** spherocylinder

EXPLANATION   A toric lens is a spherocylinder lens and is used to correct astigmatism. A spherical lens is a plus or minus lens that corrects hyperopia/presbyopia and myopia respectively.

Vertex (distance) is the length from the back surface of the eyeglass lens to the front surface of the cornea. A prism lens corrects ocular misalignment (paralytic strabismus). (Newmark 2006, 62)

9 What geometric term refers to the clearest image between the 2 focal points of a spherocylinder lens?

    a. refractive index
    b. circle of least confusion
    c. principal meridian
    d. add

ANSWER **b.** circle of least confusion

EXPLANATION The spherocylinder has 2 perpendicular radii of curvature and does not focus light to a point but to 2 lines in different places. The clearest image in the middle of these 2 lines is referred to as *the circle of least confusion* (figure). The refractive index is the ratio of the speed of light in a vacuum to its speed through a specific substance. The principal meridians are the meridians of maximum and minimum corneal curvature. The add is the part of the multifocal lens (usually the lower portion of the lens) that provides correction for near vision. (Newmark 2006, 62–63)

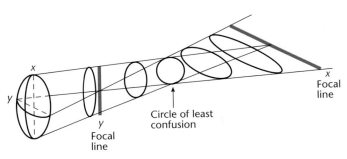

Refraction by a spherocylinder. (Reproduced, with permission, from Newmark E, ed. *Ophthalmic Medical Assisting: An Independent Study Course,* 4th ed. San Francisco: American Academy of Ophthalmology; 2006.)

10 The focal point of light rays in the figure represents an eye with what refractive error?

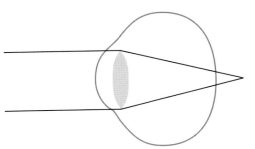

(Reproduced, with permission, from Newmark E, *Ophthalmic Medical Assisting: An Independent Study Course,* 4th ed, American Academy of Ophthalmology, 2006.)

    a. myopia
    b. hyperopia
    c. presbyopia
    d. emmetropia

ANSWER   **b.** hyperopia

EXPLANATION   In hyperopia, the cornea and lens have too little plus power for the length of the non-accommodating eye. As a result, light rays from a distant object come to a focus at a point theoretically behind the retina. In myopia, the light rays focus in front of the retina. Presbyopia is the aging eye's diminished ability to accommodate for near vision. In emmetropia, the light rays focus on the retina (normal eye). (Newmark 2006, 58)

11   What is the diopter power of a convex lens with a focal length of 40 centimeters?
   a. +5.00 D
   b. +1.00 D
   c. +0.20 D
   d. +2.50 D

ANSWER   **d.** +2.50 D

EXPLANATION   To determine the diopter power of a convex lens, the equation $D = 1/F$ must be used, where D = lens power in diopters and F = focal length in meters. Therefore, when $D = 1/0.40$ meters, $D = 2.50$ D. (Hint: 100 centimeters = 1 meter.) (Newmark 2006, 57)

12   All of the following **except** which step are part of refractometry?
   a. refinement
   b. binocular balance
   c. transposition
   d. retinoscopy

ANSWER   **c.** transposition

EXPLANATION   *Transposition* refers to converting one convention of writing an eyeglass prescription to another (plus-cylinder to minus-cylinder or vice versa). Transposition is not a step in refractometry. Refractometry may be divided into 3 separate steps: retinoscopy, refinement, and binocular balance. (Newmark 2006, 63)

13   Regarding a cross cylinder lens, all phrases below are correct **except** which of the following?

   a. consists of cylinders of equal power, a minus and a plus lens with their axis at 90° from each other
   b. used to refine the correct axis of the cylindrical lenses to treat astigmatism
   c. used to refine the correct power of the cylindrical lenses to treat astigmatism
   d. used to refine the correct power of the near vision lenses to treat presbyopia

ANSWER   **d.** used to refine the correct power of the near vision lenses to treat presbyopia

EXPLANATION   The cross cylinder lens (figure) is a useful tool for refining the axis and power of a cylindrical lens to correct astigmatism. It consists of 2 cylinders of equal power, a minus and a plus lens with their axis at 90° from each other. (Newmark 2006, 66)

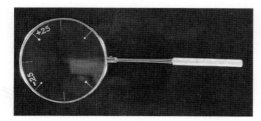

The cross cylinder, used to refine the selection of corrective cylindrical lenses for astigmatism. (Reproduced, with permission, from Newmark E, ed. *Ophthalmic Medical Assisting: An Independent Study Course,* 4th ed. San Francisco: American Academy of Ophthalmology; 2006.)

14   Refractometry includes all of the following **except** which step?

a. binocular balancing
b. lensometry
c. retinoscopy
d. refinement

ANSWER   **b.** lensometry

EXPLANATION   Although lensometry can be a useful step in measuring a patient's eyeglass prescription, it is not one of the steps of refraction. Refractometry can be divided into 3 separate steps: retinoscopy, refinement, and binocular balancing. (Newmark 2006, 63)

14 | SPECTACLE SKILLS

1   Eyeglasses with what type of lens may correct diplopia (double vision)?

a. prism lens
b. spherocylinder in each lens
c. plus lens in the dominant eye and a minus lens in the nondominant eye
d. lenses whose circle of least confusion falls on the retina in each eye

ANSWER   **a.** prism lens

EXPLANATION   Prisms are used to correct double vision. Spherocylindrical lenses are used to correct astigmatism accompanied by myopia or hyperopia. Cylindrical lenses are used to correct astigmatism. A plus lens in one eye and a minus lens in the other eye would correct farsightedness in one eye and nearsightedness in the other eye. The circle of least confusion applies to a spherical equivalent lens (a modified spherocylinder lens into only sphere power). (Newmark 2006, 62–63)

2   Which statement is correct regarding the following spectacle prescription? +2.25 +1.50 × 180 add +2.50

    a. The prescription is written for a trifocal.

    b. The prescription is for a patient with simple hyperopia.

    c. The transposed form would be +3.75 −1.50 × 90.

    d. The vertex distance needs to be included in this prescription.

ANSWER   **c.** The transposed form would be +3.75 −1.50 × 90.

EXPLANATION   Transposition of a spherocylindrical prescription involves adding the cylinder power to the spherical power, changing the sign of the cylinder power, and changing the axis by 90°. In the example, add +1.50 to +2.25, which equals +3.75. The cylinder sign changes to −1.50 and the 180 axis is changed by 90° degrees to 90°. Therefore, the transposed prescription is +3.75 −1.50 × 90. The prescription is written for a bifocal, as no intermediate power is noted. Simple hyperopia has no astigmatism in the prescription. Vertex distance is important for prescriptions with spherical power greater than plus or minus 5 diopters. (Newmark 2006, 67–68, 183–184)

3   How may transposition of an eyeglass prescription be used?

    a. to move the optical centers of the lenses away from the pupils

    b. to change the position of the bifocal in a lens

    c. to convert a minus cylinder power to a plus cylinder power

    d. to specify the distance from the eye to the back surface of the eyeglass lens

ANSWER   **c.** to convert a minus cylinder power to a plus cylinder power

EXPLANATION   Most ophthalmology offices require refractive measurements and prescriptions involving eyeglass lenses to be written in plus-cylinder form; optometrists and opticians generally use the minus-cylinder form (+ = plus or convex sphere; − = minus or concave sphere). Transposition is the mathematical conversion of a prescription written in plus cylinder form to minus cylinder form or vice-versa. Determination of the optical center and the position of the bifocal segment of eyeglass lenses are made by the dispensing optician. This does not involve transposition. The distance from the eye to the back surface of an eyeglass lens is called the *vertex power* and this is measured with a special caliper, called a *distometer*. (Newmark 2006, 68)

4   What is the correct transposition of the minus cylinder prescription +2.00 −1.00 × 180 to its plus cylinder form?

    a. +1.00 +1.00 × 180

    b. +3.00 +1.00 × 90

    c. +1.00 +1.00 × 90

    d. +2.00 +1.00 × 90

ANSWER   **c.** +1.00 +1.00 × 90

EXPLANATION   To determine the transposition of a minus cylinder prescription, first algebraically add the cylindrical power to the spherical power (−1.00 from +2.00). Then reverse the sign of the cylinder from the minus to the plus. Finally, in this case, subtract 90 from 180 to make the new axis, 90. (Newmark 2006, 68)

5   Which statement is correct regarding eyeglass frame adjustment?
  a. Optical centers should be in front of the center of the pupils.
  b. Pantoscopic tilt should be avoided.
  c. Segment height is important only for lined bi- and trifocals.
  d. Optical centers may be corrected by pantoscopic tilt.

ANSWER   a. Optical centers should be in front of the center of the pupils.

EXPLANATION   For ideal visual correction, the optical center of the eyeglass lenses must be placed directly in front of the patient's pupil. Pantoscopic tilt is routinely used. This is the angle of an eyeglass frame by which the frame front deviates from the vertical plane when the glasses are worn. This angle usually ranges from 4° to 18°. Segment height is important for both lined and progressive addition multifocal lenses. Tilting the eyeglass frame (pantoscopic tilt) does not move the position of the lens' optical center. (Newmark 2006, 73, 180, 185–188)

6   Which statement is correct regarding the base curve of an eyeglass lens?
  a. A Geneva lens clock measures only base curve of a glass lens (not plastic).
  b. The base curve is determined by the lens power.
  c. Changing base curve will not be uncomfortable if it is symmetric.
  d. The base curve is measured on the front surface of the lens.

ANSWER   d. The base curve is measured on the front surface of the lens.

EXPLANATION   The base curve is the curve of the lens surface, usually the outer or front surface of the lens, from which the other curves necessary for sign correction are calculated. A Geneva lens clock may also be used for measuring the base curve of plastic lenses. Lens clocks are calibrated for an index of refraction of 1.530. The power of a lens is determined by the algebraic difference between the power of the front curve and that of the back curve. A change in base curve from previous glasses may cause discomfort even if both the right and left lenses have the same base curve. (Newmark 2006, 184–185)

7   Which statement is correct regarding multifocal spectacle lenses?
  a. Modern progressive-addition lenses have a high patient satisfaction rate.
  b. Invisible or blended bifocals provide good intermediate-distance vision.
  c. Round top segments are increasingly popular.
  d. Patients may not change from lined to progressive-addition multifocal lenses.

ANSWER   a. Modern progressive-addition lenses have a high patient satisfaction rate.

EXPLANATION   Modern progressive lenses have a high satisfaction rate, and they have been clinically proven to work for most patients. The blended transitional zone of invisible bifocals is cosmetic and provides the wearer no area for intermediate vision. Round-top bifocals are seldom used anymore. Patients with lined multifocal eyeglass lenses may successfully change to progressive addition lenses. (Newmark 2006, 176)

8   Which statement is correct regarding eyeglass lenses?
   a. Photochromic lenses must be made of glass.
   b. Lenses may be cleaned without damage by using proper methods and materials.
   c. Polarized lenses do not protect the wearer from UVA or UVB rays.
   d. Antireflective coatings improve appearance but not vision.

ANSWER   **b.** Lenses may be cleaned without damage by using proper methods and materials.

EXPLANATION   Eyeglass lenses may be cleaned without damage by using proper methods and materials. Photochromic lenses (lenses that darken when exposed to the ultraviolet in sunlight) are available in glass and plastic. They are a good choice for all-purpose lenses. Polarized lenses protect the wearer from harmful ultraviolet rays, including ultraviolet A (UVA) and ultraviolet B (UVB) rays. By eliminating nearly all reflections from lenses, antireflective lens treatments improve appearance and vision. (Newmark 2006, 179–180, 187)

9   What type of eyeglass lenses reduce glare?
   a. tinted lenses
   b. antireflective-coated lenses
   c. photochromic lenses
   d. polarized lenses

ANSWER   **d.** polarized lenses

EXPLANATION   Only polarization of lenses truly reduce glare, and polarized lenses are available only in tinted form. Photochromic lenses and nonpolarized tinted lenses decrease light transmission through the lens, but do not eliminate glare. Antireflective-coated lenses reduce only reflections from the front and back surfaces of the lenses. These reflections are not glare; glare is reflected polarized light that comes to the observer from light-colored illuminated surfaces (ie, sunlight reflected from the surface of a body of water). (Newmark 2006, 179)

10   In most eyeglasses, the monocular pupillary distance for near vision will be less than the monocular pupillary distance for far vision by what amount?
   a. less than 1 millimeter
   b. about 2 millimeters
   c. about 4 millimeters
   d. about 6 millimeters

ANSWER   **b.** about 2 millimeters

EXPLANATION When one's eyes change from looking at a distance object to looking at a near object, the eyes have to turn in a bit (converge) so that both eyes are pointing exactly at the object that is being seen. Thus, to assure that both eyes are looking through the center of the optical correction for near, the near optical centers need to be 2 to 3 millimeters closer together than the distance optical centers in eyeglasses. If the near optical centers are not correctly positioned, the patient may experience eyestrain or even double vision when reading. (Newmark 2006, 182)

11 What is used to measure the vertex distance of a pair of eyeglasses?

  a. small millimeter ruler
  b. Geneva lens gauge
  c. caliper
  d. vertex distance comparison card

ANSWER **c.** caliper

EXPLANATION The distance from the front of the eye to the back of the eyeglass lens is measured with a caliper. Often called a *distometer*, the caliper that is calibrated to account for the thickness of the closed eyelid over which the caliper is applied. Millimeter rulers and comparison cards are subject to parallax errors. A Geneva lens gauge does not measure distance; it measures surface curves of a lens. (Newmark 2006, 183–184)

12 Which statement is correct regarding measurements used to fit eyeglasses?

  a. The base curve is the back curve of the lens surface.
  b. The near pupillary distance is required to manufacture all eyeglasses.
  c. The vertex distance is the distance from the back surface of the lens to the cornea.
  d. The optical center varies depending on vertex distance.

ANSWER **c.** The vertex distance is the distance from the back surface of the lens to the cornea.

EXPLANATION The vertex distance is the distance from the back surface of the lens to the cornea. It is used for prescriptions of 5 diopters or greater, and measured with a distometer. The base curve is the curve on the front surface of the lens. Only the distant pupillary distance is required to fabricate single vision distance glasses. The optical center is a fixed point in the lens that is not affected by the distance between the back surface of the lens and the cornea (vertex distance). (Newmark 2006, 183–184)

13 What does a Geneva lens clock measure?

  a. pantoscopic angle
  b. base curve
  c. segment height
  d. optical center

ANSWER   **b.** base curve

EXPLANATION   A Geneva lens clock is an instrument that measures the base curve of a lens. It will measure the base curve of both plastic and glass lenses. Pantoscopic tilt is the angle of an eyeglass frame by which the frame front deviates from the vertical plane when the glasses are worn. Segment height is the distance between the lowest part of an eyeglass rim and the top of the multifocal or add segment. Optical center is the single point of a lens that would provide optimal vision. (Newmark 2006, 185)

14   What is the recommended height of a bifocal segment?
   a. dissecting the pupil
   b. lower lid margin
   c. 5 mm below the lower lid
   d. 5 mm above the lower lid margin

ANSWER   **b.** lower lid margin

EXPLANATION   Most opticians recommend fitting the top of the bifocal segment level (figure) with the patient's lower lid margin. The lower lid margin is the area where the lid touches the eyeball. (Newmark 2006, 187–188)

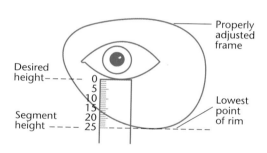

Placement of bifocal segment. (Reproduced, with permission, from Newmark E, ed. *Ophthalmic Medical Assisting: An Independent Study Course,* 4th ed. San Francisco: American Academy of Ophthalmology; 2006.)

15 SUPPLEMENTAL SKILLS

1   In measuring axial length, what is the most common cause of error?
   a. a short axial length due to compression of the cornea with contact A-scan ultrasonography
   b. a poor echo due to a dry cornea when measuring with contact A-scan ultrasonography
   c. a short axial length due to compression of the sclera by the immersion scan shell
   d. a long axial length due to an off-axis scan with immersion A-scan ultrasonography

ANSWER   **a.** a short axial length due to compression of the cornea with contact A-scan ultrasonography

EXPLANATION   The most common cause of error in measuring axial length is a falsely short axial length due to compression of the cornea in contact A-scan ultrasonography. For this reason, some consider immersion A-scan ultrasonography to be more accurate, as corneal compression cannot occur with this noncontact method. (Stein 2006, 517)

2   What is the test called that places a strip of filter paper in the outer lower fornix of the eye?

    a. gonioscopy
    b. corneal sensitivity
    c. Schirmer
    d. Worth 4-dot

ANSWER   **c.** Schirmer

EXPLANATION   A Schirmer test determines the tear output produced in 5 minutes and helps the ophthalmologist in the diagnosis of a dry eye condition. Gonioscopy is a test to visualize the angle of the eye to determine any change that may contribute to glaucoma. The corneal sensitivity test, done with a thin cotton wisp touching the unanesthetized cornea, helps determine diseases that result in the loss of normal corneal sensitivity. The Worth 4-dot test is used to measure the alignment of the eye. (Newmark 2006, 135)

3   What is the minimal tear-film breakup time considered normal?

    a. 3 seconds
    b. 6 seconds
    c. 10 seconds
    d. 30 seconds

ANSWER   **c.** 10 seconds

EXPLANATION   A normal tear-film breakup time (TBUT) is at least 10 seconds. (Patel 2003, 27; Stein 2006, 819)

4   What is the average axial length of the human eye?

    a. 21.00 to 22.00 mm
    b. 23.00 to 23.50 mm
    c. 25.00 to 26.00 mm
    d. 26.00 to 28.00 mm

ANSWER   **b.** 23.00 to 23.50 mm

EXPLANATION   Axial length is measured from the front of the cornea to the fovea. The average axial length is 23.00 to 23.50 mm. The axial length is part of the information necessary to calculate the appropriate intraocular lens implant power. (Kendall 1991, 161)

5   What is the normal thickness of the central cornea?

    a. 0.47 mm
    b. 0.56 mm
    c. 0.61 mm
    d. 0.68 mm

ANSWER   **b.** 0.56 mm

EXPLANATION   Average central corneal thickness is 0.56 to 0.58 mm. The peripheral cornea is thicker, approximately 1 mm thick. A thicker or thinner central cornea affects the measurement reading of a Goldmann applanation tonometer. A thicker cornea intraocular pressure measurement will be higher than expected and thinner vice versa. (Newmark 2006, 36, 144)

6   To estimate the anterior chamber depth, what is the first step?

    a. Shine a flashlight near the limbus from the temporal side of the eye.
    b. Shine a flashlight near the limbus from the nasal side of the eye.
    c. Shine a flashlight into the eye at an angle of 45°.
    d. Shine a flashlight directly into the eye.

ANSWER   **a.** Shine a flashlight near the limbus from the temporal side of the eye.

EXPLANATION   The flashlight test for anterior chamber depth is performed by shining a flashlight or transilluminator from the temporal side near the limbus (figure). This simple test screens for the presence of a shallow anterior chamber. The other options will not create the result desired. (Newmark 2006, 132–133)

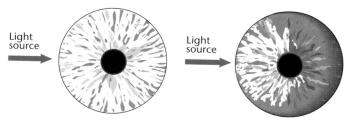

Performing the flashlight test to estimate anterior depth. Left: In an eye with a normally shaped anterior chamber and iris, the nasal half of the iris will be illuminated like the temporal half. Right: In an eye with a shallow anterior chamber and narrow chamber angle, about two-thirds of the nasal portion of the iris will appear in shadow. (Reproduced, with permission, from Newmark E, ed. *Ophthalmic Medical Assisting: An Independent Study Course,* 4th ed. San Francisco: American Academy of Ophthalmology; 2006.)

7   Gonioscopy is used to examine which of the following?

    a. retina
    b. lens
    c. angle structure of the eye
    d. conjunctiva

ANSWER   **c.** angle structure of the eye

EXPLANATION   Gonioscopy is an exam of the anterior chamber and angle structures of the eye. This exam helps to differentiate between open-angle and narrow-angle glaucoma. (Newmark 2006, 133–134)

8   What is a normal tear production measurement for a Schirmer test with topical anesthetic (Schirmer II)?

    a. more than 10 mm in 5 minutes
    b. more than 5 mm in 10 minutes
    c. more than 15 mm in 15 minutes
    d. more than 10 mm in 10 minutes

ANSWER   **a.** more than 10 mm in 5 minutes

EXPLANATION   Normal tear production for a Schirmer test with topical anesthetic wets at least 10 mm of the filter paper strip over a period of 5 minutes. (Newmark 2006, 135)

9   What does the phenol red thread test measure?

    a. color vision
    b. ocular pH
    c. corneal sensitivity
    d. tear output

ANSWER   **d.** tear output

EXPLANATION   The phenol red thread test is similar to the Schirmer test and measures tear output. Color vision is most commonly tested with pseudoisochromatic color plates. Clinically, corneal sensation is tested with a sterile wisp of cotton. Ocular pH test does not exist. (Newmark 2006, 136)

10   Increased corneal thickness is commonly associated with which of the following?

    a. pingueculitis
    b. abnormalities of the corneal endothelial cells
    c. abnormalities of the corneal epithelial cells
    d. scleritis and episcleritis

ANSWER   **b.** abnormalities of the corneal endothelial cells

EXPLANATION   There are 5 layers of the cornea (figure). Corneal thickness commonly increases when there are abnormalities of the endothelial cells of the cornea. The endothelial cells are responsible for removing fluid from the corneal stroma, keeping it relatively dehydrated. When the endothelial cells fail, the cornea becomes edematous (swollen), increasing in thickness and becoming hazy. Pingueculitis is an inflammation of a pinguecula (a thickened yellowish area on the bulbar conjunctiva) and is not associated with corneal swelling. The corneal epithelium is the front barrier surface of the cornea and has limited function in maintaining corneal dehydration. Scleritis and episcleritis are inflammatory conditions that are not associated with increased corneal thickness. (Newmark 2006, 144)

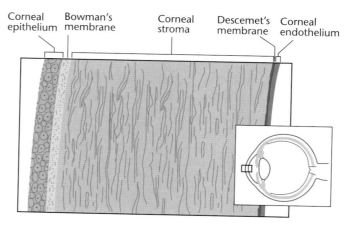

The 5 layers of the cornea. (Reproduced, with permission, from Newmark E, ed. *Ophthalmic Medical Assisting: An Independent Study Course,* 4th ed. San Francisco: American Academy of Ophthalmology; 2006.)

11   How are ultrasonography units calibrated?

    a. by touching the probe to a test block specific for that machine
    b. by touching the probe to a flat surface
    c. by routinely measuring the same person's eye as a standard
    d. by pressing the instrument calibration button

ANSWER   **a.** by touching the probe to a test block specific for that machine

EXPLANATION   Manufacturers of ultrasonography (biometric) instruments provide a standardized test block or model eye to test the accuracy of their instrument. Measurements are taken while the probe is touching the test block. The ophthalmic medical assistant does the measurement after checking the calibration of the instrument. For more information, refer to the manufacturer's operation manual for the specific instrument in your office.

12   A 65-year-old patient has the sensation of a foreign body in her eyes, as well as tearing and blurring of the eyes, especially in windy situations. What test would be most helpful for this patient?

    a. pinhole test
    b. indirect ophthalmoscopy
    c. Schirmer test
    d. visual field test

ANSWER   **c.** Schirmer test

EXPLANATION   The patient's complaints are consistent with dry eye symptoms, and the test that is most helpful measures the tear output, which is the Schirmer test. This test may be done with topical anesthetic (measures basic secretion) or without topical anesthetic (measures reflex tearing). The pinhole test is done during vision assessment of an individual with less than 20/20 vision. Indirect ophthalmoscopy is performed by the ophthalmologist to examine the retina. The visual field test is performed to assess the boundaries of the patient's peripheral vision. (Newmark 2006, 135)

13   Most patients tested for glare sensitivity with the brightness acuity tester (BAT) have significant decrease in vision at what light intensity?

    a. low-medium
    b. medium
    c. medium-high
    d. high

ANSWER   **b.** medium

EXPLANATION   Glare testing assesses the patient's vision in the presence of a bright light to determine if the sensitivity to glare is contributing to the patient's visual symptoms. A common device is the brightness acuity tester (figure). This instrument has 3 settings to simulate a variety of lighting conditions: a low setting simulates a brightly lit room; a medium setting, outdoor sunlight; and a high setting, sunlight reflected off concrete, beach sand, or water. Most patients have significant decrease in vision at the medium intensity. (Newmark 2006, 143–144)

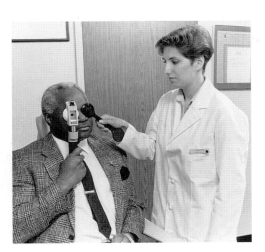

Glare testing. (Reproduced, with permission, from Newmark E, ed. *Ophthalmic Medical Assisting: An Independent Study Course,* 4th ed. San Francisco: American Academy of Ophthalmology; 2006.)

14   What information is necessary to calculate the power of an intraocular lens?

    a. corneal thickness, axial length, and lens manufacturer's A constant
    b. corneal diameter, axial length, and lens manufacturer's A constant
    c. corneal curvature, patient's refractive error, lens manufacturer's A constant
    d. corneal curvature, axial length, and lens manufacturer's A constant

ANSWER   **d.** corneal curvature, axial length, and lens manufacturer's A constant

EXPLANATION   To calculate the appropriate power of the intraocular lens (IOL), you need the corneal curvature measurement (keratometry reading), axial length (A-scan measurement), and the manufacturer's A constant of the lens (found in the package insert). Corneal thickness is not used in IOL power calculations, although it is important for glaucoma patients. Corneal diameter is also not used in IOL power calculation, but it is important for estimating the length of anteriorly placed IOLs. The patient's refractive error prior to developing a cataract is important information that can be used to help support the final calculated IOL power, but it is not required for the calculation. (Newmark 2006, 145, 147–148; Stein 2006, 517)

15   Which of the following will result from a 1-mm error in axial length measurement?

a. approximately 3 D of change in postoperative refractive error
b. approximately 2 D of change in postoperative refractive error
c. approximately 1 D of change in postoperative refractive error
d. no significant change in postoperative refractive error

ANSWER   a. approximately 3 D of change in postoperative refractive error

EXPLANATION   An axial length of 1 mm is approximately equal to 3 D of change in refractive error. Knowing that such an error can alter the patient's final postoperative correction highlights the importance of accurate and skillful biometry. (Newmark 2006, 147; Stein 2006, 517)

16   Which device is used to measure corneal thickness?

a. tonometer
b. keratometer
c. phoropter
d. pachymeter

ANSWER   d. pachymeter

EXPLANATION   A pachymeter measures corneal thickness. A tonometer measures intraocular pressure, a keratometer measures corneal curvature, and a phoropter is used to determine a patient's refractive error subjectively. (Newmark 2006, 144)

17   Which statement is **incorrect** regarding anterior chamber depth?

a. It is often shallower in a patient with nuclear sclerotic cataracts.
b. It is usually shallower in a patient with myopia than in a patient with hyperopia.
c. It may affect intraocular pressure.
d. It can be compressed when a contact A-scan probe is used.

ANSWER   b. It is usually shallower in a patient with myopia than in a patient with hyperopia.

EXPLANATION　As nuclear sclerotic cataracts develop, the crystalline lens thickens, pushing forward slightly and shallowing the anterior chamber depth. A hyperopic (farsighted) eye is typically smaller, with a shorter axial length and shallower anterior chamber, than a myopic (nearsighted) eye. A shallow anterior chamber has a narrower angle. This may lead to reduced aqueous outflow and increased intraocular pressure. As a contact A-scan measurement is being performed, it compresses the cornea, which shortens the anterior chamber measurement. (Newmark 2006, 18, 36, 132; Stein 2006, 171–173, 517)

16 | TONOMETRY

1　The examiner is preparing to measure intraocular pressure with the Goldmann applanation tonometer. Which of the following must be instilled into the eye, along with the topical anesthetic?

  a. rose bengal
  b. fluorescein
  c. lissamine green
  d. gentian violet

ANSWER　**b.** fluorescein

EXPLANATION　Topical anesthetic is required for applanation tonometry. The procedure is performed using the blue light on the slit lamp and with fluorescein dye instilled in the eye. (Newmark 2006, 129–130)

2　In the measurement of intraocular pressure (IOP) with the Goldmann applanation tonometer, the intraocular pressure is indicated by a number on the calibrated dial. This reading is multiplied by what number to express the IOP in millimeters of mercury?

  a. 2
  b. 5
  c. 10
  d. 20

ANSWER　**c.** 10

EXPLANATION　The figure shows the Goldmann tonometer. The tonometer tip is applied to the cornea, and the force is increased by turning the force adjustment knob until a circle of cornea 3.06 mm in diameter is flattened. The amount of force required is indicated by a number on the calibrated dial on the adjustment knob. This reading is simply multiplied by 10. (Newmark 2006, 129)

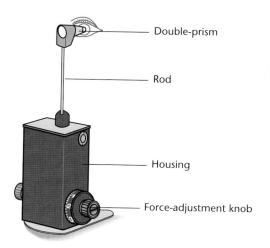

Double-prism

Rod

Housing

Force-adjustment knob

The Goldmann applanation tonometer.
(Reproduced, with permission, from Newmark
E, ed. *Ophthalmic Medical Assisting:
An Independent Study Course,* 4th ed.
San Francisco: American Academy of
Ophthalmology, 2006.)

3   A patient undergoing Goldmann tonometry has a central corneal thickness significantly thicker than average. What can be said of the endpoint shown in the figure?

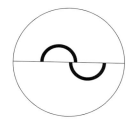

(Reproduced, with permission, from Newmark E, ed. *Ophthalmic Medical
Assisting: An Independent Study Course,* 4th ed. San Francisco: American
Academy of Ophthalmology; 2006.)

a. It is correct, but the reading is significantly higher than the actual intraocular pressure.
b. It is correct, but the reading is significantly lower than the actual intraocular pressure.
c. It is incorrect, and the examiner should adjust the knob so that the mires are spread apart.
d. It is incorrect, and the examiner should adjust the knob so that the mires are closer together.

ANSWER   **a.** It is correct, but the reading is significantly higher than the actual intraocular pressure.

EXPLANATION   Corneal thickness has no effect on the endpoint achieved when taking a reading with the Goldmann applanation tonometer. The endpoint shown is correct with the hemicircles just touching on the inside. However, a thicker-than-average cornea will require extra force to achieve the endpoint, resulting in overestimation of the intraocular pressure. (Newmark 2006, 127–130)

4   What is a way the air-puff tonometer differs from the Goldmann tonometer?
a. It is an indentation tonometer.
b. It uses a red stain on the cornea.
c. It is a noncontact approach.
d. It always reads lower.

ANSWER   **c.** It is a noncontact approach.

EXPLANATION   The air-puff tonometer is the classic noncontact tonometer. It employs a burst of air to applanate the cornea. Therefore, it is not an indention tonometer, needs no dye or anesthetic, and the readings are quite accurate. (Newmark 2006, 129)

5   What is a disadvantage of the Goldman applanation tonometer?
   a. It is not standardized.
   b. It is not portable.
   c. It is hard to sterilize.
   d. Reproducibility of readings is poor.

ANSWER   **b.** It is not portable.

EXPLANATION   The Goldmann tonometer must be mounted on a slit lamp in order to be used. The calibration and use of the instrument are highly standardized, reproducibility is high (1 mm Hg), and the tips are easily cleaned and sterilized. (Newmark 2006, 129)

6   What is a potential disadvantage of using the Schiøtz tonometer in a highly myopic eye?
   a. The patient will squint because the instrument is in focus as it approaches the eye.
   b. Myopic eyes are prone to corneal abrasions from the tip.
   c. Intraocular pressure will be underestimated due to low scleral rigidity.
   d. Intraocular pressure will be overestimated due to high scleral rigidity.

ANSWER   **c.** Intraocular pressure will be underestimated due to low scleral rigidity.

EXPLANATION   The "elastic" myopic eye wall will dissipate the applied weight and not push back on the instrument with the full force of the intraocular pressure, resulting in underestimation of the pressure. (Newmark 2006, 131–132)

7   How should the plastic tip of an applanation tonometer be cleaned after use?
   a. wiped with a clean tissue
   b. soaked in 5% boric acid solution for 5 minutes, rinsed, and allowed to dry
   c. soaked in a 1:10 solution of household bleach, rinsed, and allowed to dry
   d. boiled for 3 minutes in sterile water

ANSWER   **c.** soaked in a 1:10 solution of household bleach, rinsed, and allowed to dry

EXPLANATION   There are several techniques for cleaning a tonometer tip after use, such as wiping the entire tip with an alcohol sponge and allowing it to air-dry. Wiping with a clean tissue is not adequate, however. A germicide must be used to insure that infectious agents, particularly viruses, are killed. Soaking the tip in 3% hydrogen peroxide or a 1:10 solution of household bleach for 5 minutes, then rinsing with water before replacing the tip on the biomicroscope is a required technique. A boric acid solution is not recommended, nor is boiling, both of which could damage the fragile tip and the prism inside. (Newmark 2006, 294)

8 Which of the following variables can affect an applanation tonometry measurement?

a. height of the patient
b. gender of the patient
c. corneal thickness
d. anterior chamber depth

ANSWER c. corneal thickness

EXPLANATION Applanation tonometry measures intraocular pressure by analyzing the force required to flatten a small area of the central cornea. Corneal thickness affects the readings: thick corneas measure falsely higher pressure and thin corneas measure falsely lower pressure: the patient's height and gender do not affect the measurement, nor does the anterior chamber depth alone. (Newmark 2006, 127)

9 A patient is tending to squeeze the eye shut during applanation tonometry. Which of the following is most likely to result in satisfactory pressure readings?

a. Explain to the patient the importance of keeping the eye open.
b. Insert a speculum to keep the eye open.
c. Hold both eyelids open with one hand.
d. Use a cotton-tipped applicator to gently elevate the upper eyelid.

ANSWER d. Use a cotton-tipped applicator to gently elevate the upper eyelid.

EXPLANATION Elevating the upper eyelid while avoiding pressure on the globe, using your thumb or a cotton-tipped applicator, is the best way to obtain accurate readings. (Newmark 2006, 130)

10 Which of the following has **no** effect upon the intraocular pressure reading obtained with the Goldmann applanation tonometer?

a. corneal astigmatism
b. corneal thickness
c. external pressure on the eye from the examiner's fingers
d. a tight collar or necktie

ANSWER a. corneal astigmatism

EXPLANATION Corneal astigmatism has no effect upon the intraocular pressure. A thinner than average cornea will result in lower pressure readings than the actual pressure and vice versa for a thicker cornea. External pressure or anything that impedes venous drainage from the head, such as a tight collar or necktie, will elevate the pressure readings. (Newmark 2006, 128–130)

11   Which of the following tonometers does **not** provide a direct pressure reading in mm Hg?

a. Schiøtz tonometer
b. Goldmann tonometer
c. Tono-Pen tonometer
d. Air-puff tonometer

ANSWER   a. Schiøtz tonometer

EXPLANATION   The Schiøtz tonometer measures indentation of the cornea by the applied weight. The number on the scale corresponds to a mm Hg measurement obtained from a conversion table based upon the scale reading and the applied weight. All of the other instruments provide a direct reading in mm Hg. (Newmark 2006, 131–132)

12   If the upper eyelid is resting on the applanation tonometer tip (unaware to the examiner), which of the following is **not** likely?

a. The pressure will be underestimated.
b. The pressure will be overestimated.
c. An accurate reading will be obtained.
d. The mires will be distorted.

ANSWER   c. An accurate reading will be obtained.

EXPLANATION   It is unlikely to obtain an accurate reading with the eyelid resting on the tip. All of the others are possible. (Newmark 2006, 130)

13   Which of the following is **not** an applanation tonometer?

a. Tono-Pen tonometer
b. Perkins tonometer
c. MacKay-Marg tonometer
d. Schiøtz tonometer

ANSWER   d. Schiøtz tonometer

EXPLANATION   The Schiøtz tonometer is an indentation tonometer. The other tonometers listed are based on applanation. (Newmark 2006, 129–131)

17 VISUAL ASSESSMENT

1   What is the first procedure performed during the physical examination of a patient's eyes?

    a.   discussion of the reason the patient has come to the ophthalmologist's office (chief complaint)
    b.   measurement of visual acuity
    c.   measurement of the intraocular pressure
    d.   examination of the pupillary response

ANSWER   **b.**   measurement of visual acuity

EXPLANATION   Visual acuity (VA) is always the first test to be completed. The chief complaint is part of history taking and not part of the physical examination. The intraocular pressure (IOP) measurement is performed after the VA measurement. Once the IOP is measured, the VA may no longer be accurate because the surface of the cornea may become irregular. The pupillary exam is performed after the VA measurement. Once a light has been shined into the eye, a recovery period may be necessary before an accurate VA can be determined. (Newmark 2006, 112)

2   What does a pinhole acuity test confirm?

    a.   The patient has a vitreous hemorrhage that is causing below-normal vision.
    b.   The patient is legally blind.
    c.   The patient is presbyopic.
    d.   The patient has a refractive error that is the cause of below-normal vision.

ANSWER   **d.**   The patient has a refractive error that is the cause of below-normal vision.

EXPLANATION   The pinhole acuity test confirms whether a refractive error is the cause of below-normal visual acuity. The patient views the Snellen acuity chart through a pinhole occluder. The pinhole admits only parallel rays of light that does not require focusing by the eye, thus the patient is able to resolve fine detail on the visual acuity chart without an optical correction. A vitreous hemorrhage is confirmed by a dilated examination. Legal blindness is 20/200 vision or less, and is confirmed by a proper refraction. Presbyopia, the loss of accommodative ability by the lens due to aging, is confirmed by a patient's birth date and symptoms. (Newmark 2006, 119)

3   Near vision is measured at what distance from the patient's eyes, unless specifically recorded otherwise?

    a.   6 inches
    b.   10 inches
    c.   14 inches
    d.   18 inches

ANSWER   **c.**   14 inches

EXPLANATION   While any measured distance can be used for near acuity testing, 14 inches is the testing standard. If using any other test distance, the tester must record the distance used in the record (for example, J4 at 6 inches). (Newmark 2006, 119–121)

4   Which of the following is a measure for visual acuity?

    a. the ability to see traffic clearly when driving a car
    b. the ability to read
    c. a Snellen chart
    d. the ability to follow a golf ball once hit

ANSWER   **c.** a Snellen chart

EXPLANATION   The ability to read, follow a golf ball once hit, and see traffic clearly when driving are all abilities of visual function, but they are not measurements of visual acuity. The Snellen chart (figure) is the standard for measuring distance visual acuity. (Newmark 2006, 117)

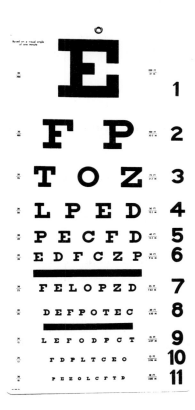

The Snellen chart used for testing distance visual acuity. (Reproduced, with permission, from Newmark E, ed. *Ophthalmic Medical Assisting: An Independent Study Course,* 4th ed. San Francisco: American Academy of Ophthalmology; 2006.)

5   Visual acuity of 20/40 indicates that the patient sees which of the following?

    a. at 20 feet what a normal eye would see at 40 feet
    b. at 40 feet what a normal eye would see at 20 feet
    c. at 20 feet what a normal eye would see at 20 feet
    d. at 40 feet what a normal eye would see at 40 feet

ANSWER   **a.** at 20 feet what a normal eye would see at 40 feet

EXPLANATION   The first number in the Snellen notation indicates the distance at which the test is performed. The second number is the distance from which a normal eye could see that size letter. Occasionally moving the patient closer to the Snellen acuity chart may be helpful for patients with reduced vision—15, 10, or 5 feet, thereby changing the first number in the Snellen notation (10/20). However, moving the chart further from the patient (>20 feet) is never employed. (Newmark 2006, 117–119, 231)

6   Using the metric system, a vision of 6/24 is the same as which of the following?

    a. 20/24 in the English system
    b. 20/6 in the English system
    c. 20/60 in the English system
    d. 20/80 in the English system

ANSWER   **d.** 20/80 in the English system

EXPLANATION   Distance vision can be recorded in meters (m) where 6 m = 20 feet. In this example, the patient standing at 6 m could read only the 24 m letter size that a normal eye could read at 24 m (4 times closer than a patient with normal vision). To convert to the English system, divide the second number by 6 (24 ÷ 6 = 4) then multiply the result (4) by 20 = 20/80. (Newmark 2006, 118)

7   What does the term *ocular media* refer to?

    a. the average vision considering both eyes
    b. the cornea and the retina
    c. a cataract
    d. the cornea, lens, and vitreous

ANSWER   **d.** the cornea, lens, and vitreous

EXPLANATION   The ocular media include all of the transparent structures in the eye: the cornea, lens, and vitreous. Sometimes the aqueous is included as well. A cataract is an opacity of the lens. The average vision of both eyes is not a useful clinical measurement and is unrelated to the ocular media. The cornea is part of the ocular media but the retina is not a transparent structure of the eye. (Newmark 2006, 142)

8   Which phrase is accurate regarding cataract removal with intraocular lens implantation?

    a. is rarely performed
    b. can often restore vision to an excellent level
    c. is contraindicated with a dense white cataract
    d. is contraindicated to perform as an outpatient

ANSWER   **b.** can often restore vision to an excellent level

EXPLANATION   Cataract surgery with intraocular lens implantation is the most frequently performed ocular operation and regularly restores excellent vision. The surgery is usually performed as an outpatient and a dense, white cataract is not a contraindication for surgery. (Newmark 2006, 142)

9   Which of the following can affect the clarity of the cornea?

   a. scars and edema
   b. temporal arteritis
   c. cataract
   d. amblyopia

ANSWER   **a.** scars and edema

EXPLANATION   Corneal scars and corneal edema decrease the clarity of the cornea. A cataract is an opacity of the lens. Temporal arteritis is an inflammation of arteries that can lead to loss of vision and is a true ocular emergency. Amblyopia ("lazy eye") is decreased vision resulting from visual deprivation in early childhood. (Newmark 2006, 142)

10   Which phrase accurately describes corneal transplantation?

   a. often restores excellent vision in patients with no light perception (NLP) vision
   b. often restores excellent vision in patients with corneal scars
   c. cannot restore vision in patient's with corneal edema
   d. should not be performed in the elderly

ANSWER   **b.** often restores excellent vision in patients with corneal scars

EXPLANATION   Corneal transplantation is a very successful procedure in young and old adults with corneal scars. Patients with NLP vision will not benefit from a corneal transplant. Excellent results may also be obtained in patients with corneal edema. (Newmark 2006, 142)

11   Which phrase is correct regarding visual potential tests?

   a. are an alternate method of measuring visual acuity
   b. grade the density of a cataract
   c. bypass opacities in the ocular media to measure the visual potential of the retina and optic nerve
   d. are inaccurate and should not be performed

ANSWER   **c.** bypass opacities in the ocular media to measure the visual potential of the retina and optic nerve

EXPLANATION   Visual potential tests are very helpful in counseling patients regarding the visual result they can expect after surgery to correct obstructions in the ocular media, such as cataract removal and corneal transplants. They do not measure current visual acuity or grade the density of a cataract. (Newmark 2006, 142)

12   What phrase applies to the potential acuity meter (PAM)?

  a. projects a Snellen acuity chart through a window in the media opacity
  b. must be performed with the pupil dilated
  c. works in cases of cataract but not for corneal scarring
  d. is rarely useful

ANSWER   **a.** projects a Snellen acuity chart through a window in the media opacity

EXPLANATION   The PAM (figure) is frequently useful in approximating the postoperative vision in patients who have opacities of the media and concurrent abnormalities of the retina or optic nerve. It may work better through a dilated pupil, but this is not necessary. It projects a Snellen acuity chart onto the retina through a window in the opacity, thereby measuring the visual potential of the retina and optic nerve. (Newmark 2006, 142)

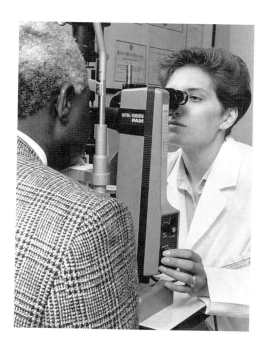

Testing with a potential acuity meter (PAM). (Reproduced, with permission, from Newmark E, ed. *Ophthalmic Medical Assisting: An Independent Study Course,* 4th ed. San Francisco: American Academy of Ophthalmology; 2006.)

13   Which phrase applies to contrast sensitivity testing?

  a. is unimportant
  b. is an important, but difficult part of the visual assessment
  c. is important, and can be determined in an office setting
  d. requires expensive and difficult-to-use equipment

ANSWER   **c.** is important, and can be determined in an office setting

EXPLANATION   Patients may be able to perform well on Snellen visual acuity testing, but they still have significant and important visual problems. Contrast sensitivity testing can be performed in an office setting with specialized charts easily and inexpensively (figure). (Newmark 2006, 143)

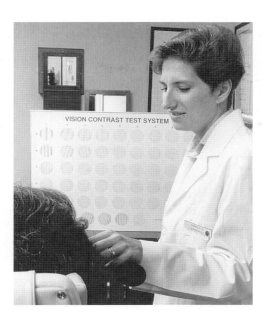

Contrast-sensitivity testing. (Reproduced, with permission, from Newmark E, ed. *Ophthalmic Medical Assisting: An Independent Study Course,* 4th ed. San Francisco: American Academy of Ophthalmology, 2006.)

14   Which phrase applies to the brightness acuity tester (BAT)?

    a. is another way to test potential vision
    b. is another way to measure best corrected visual acuity
    c. is a method of demonstrating a patient's complaint regarding decreased visual acuity in bright light
    d. determines whether a cataract operation will be successful

ANSWER   **c.** is a method of demonstrating a patient's complaint regarding decreased visual acuity in bright light

EXPLANATION   The BAT is a glare tester that determines how light glare affects the patient's vision. The BAT requires the patient to read the Snellen chart through a translucent cup that can be illuminated with 3 different levels of light. Patients with significant cataracts will sometimes do surprisingly well on standard Snellen acuity testing, but they will have a significant decrease in visual acuity testing with the BAT at medium illumination. It does not test potential vision or best corrected visual acuity (quite the opposite) and cannot predict the results of cataract surgery. (Newmark 2006, 144)

15   Which of the following statements applies to infants and young children?

    a. They cannot have their vision assessed.
    b. They should have their eyes tested quickly.
    c. They require patience when being examined for visual assessment.
    d. They should wait until they know the alphabet before seeing an ophthalmologist.

ANSWER   **c.** They require patience when being examined for visual assessment.

EXPLANATION   Infants have the ability to follow objects or light and young children have the ability to identify pictures. These tests help to determine the level of their visual perception. Speed in testing vision in young children is to be avoided. The ability to read letters or numbers is not essential to assess a basic level of vision in infants and young children. (Newmark 2006, 231–234)

16   How should near acuity be measured?

   a. without a lens in front of the eye and the near card held at 14 inches
   b. with both eyes opened and reading a book in good lighting
   c. monocularly with the distance correction with additional plus power lens
   d. with a + 2.50 lens for each eye holding a near card at 14 inches

ANSWER   **c.** monocularly with the distance correction with additional plus power lens

EXPLANATION   Near acuity is measured for each eye individually best corrected for distance with the addition of a plus power lens appropriate for the patient's age, and the near card or an eye chart that has letters sized to be held at 14 inches. (Newmark 2006, 119–121)

18 | VISUAL FIELDS

1   What is the term for an area of reduced sensitivity in the visual field?

   a. isopter
   b. scotoma
   c. boundary
   d. contour

ANSWER   **b.** scotoma

EXPLANATION   A scotoma by definition is an area of reduced visual sensitivity. An isopter is not a measure of reduced sensitivity. It is rather a circular boundary around an area of sensitivity. A boundary and contour are not measurements of sensitivity. (Newmark 2006, 158)

2   The Amsler grid would be most helpful for a patient with which of the following?

   a. cataract
   b. glaucoma
   c. retinal detachment
   d. macular degeneration

ANSWER   **d.** macular degeneration

EXPLANATION   The Amsler grid tests the central visual field. The grid is used to detect visual changes in patients with macular pathology, most commonly macular degeneration. Cataract is evaluated by visual assessment, slit-lamp exam, and glare testing. Glaucoma is evaluated by intraocular pressure, optic disc, and visual field studies. Retinal detachment is evaluated by visual assessment, visual field test, and fundus exam. (Newmark 2006, 126, 128)

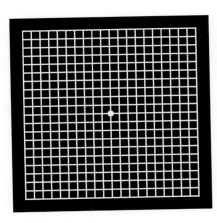

The Amsler grid test. The typical white-on-black Amsler grid. (Reproduced, with permission, from Newmark E, ed. *Ophthalmic Medical Assisting: An Independent Study Course,* 4th ed. San Francisco: American Academy of Ophthalmology; 2006.)

3   The center of the island of vision corresponds to what part of the eye?

    a. lens
    b. iris
    c. pupil
    d. fovea

ANSWER   **d.** fovea

EXPLANATION   The figure shows locations within the retina. The most sensitive anatomical retinal area is the fovea. The lens, iris, and pupil are not visual receptors. The lens is involved in focusing light onto the retina. The iris is the color part of the eye behind the cornea, and the pupil is the opening in the iris through which light passes. (Newmark 2006, 154)

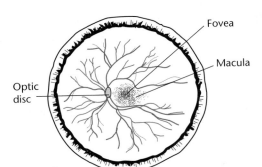

Locations within the retina. (Reproduced, with permission, from Newmark E, ed. *Ophthalmic Medical Assisting: An Independent Study Course,* 4th ed. San Francisco: American Academy of Ophthalmology; 2006.)

4   The visual information travels from the optic tracts to terminate in which part of the brain?

    a. frontal lobe
    b. temporal lobe
    c. parietal lobe
    d. occipital lobe

ANSWER   **d.** occipital lobe

EXPLANATION   The pathway of vision commences in the retina, then travels in the optic nerve to the optic chiasm and from there through the optic tracts to the occipital lobe via the optic radiations (figure). The frontal lobe is anterior to the tracts and radiations and is not part of the visual pathway. The temporal lobe and parietal lobe are involved as a conduit in the visual pathway for the optic radiations. The visual information terminates in the occipital lobe. (Newmark 2006, 154)

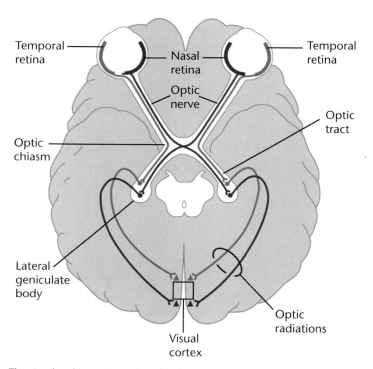

The visual pathway. (Reproduced, with permission, from Newmark E, ed. *Ophthalmic Medical Assisting: An Independent Study Course,* 4th ed. San Francisco: American Academy of Ophthalmology; 2006.)

5   In what direction is the largest boundary of a normal visual field?

    a. temporally
    b. nasally
    c. superiorly
    d. inferiorly

ANSWER   **a.** temporally

EXPLANATION   The figure shows boundaries of a normal visual field. The largest visual field is temporal. The forehead blocks the superior field, the nose blocks the medial field, and the maxilla blocks the inferior field from having a full field. The temporal field may extend to 90° or more. The superior and nasal fields' extent is an angle of about 60°. The inferior field extends an angle of about 70°. (Newmark 2006, 156)

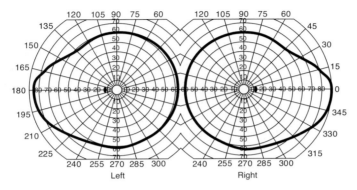

Boundaries of a normal visual field. The black spot in the temporal field of each eye represents the physiologic blind spot. (Reproduced, with permission, from Newmark E, ed. *Ophthalmic Medical Assisting: An Independent Study Course,* 4th ed. San Francisco: American Academy of Ophthalmology; 2006.)

6   What is the purpose of perimetry?

a. to detect abnormalities in the visual field
b. to detect cataractous changes
c. to follow progression of a third cranial nerve palsy
d. to diagnose congenital color defects

ANSWER   **a.** to detect abnormalities in the visual field

EXPLANATION   Perimetry maps the shape of the patient's visual field and any defects within it. It is crucial to the diagnosis and monitoring of a variety of ophthalmic conditions, especially those affecting the retina, optic nerve, and visual pathway. A visual field test can show defects that are not observed by the patient. Cataractous changes can be followed with changes in the patient's vision or by direct observation with the slit lamp. Third cranial nerve palsy, a condition caused by damage to the oculomotor nerve, is monitored by clinical evaluation and neurovascular imaging. Congenital color defects are diagnosed through pseudoisochromatic color plates or more extensive color vision testing. (Newmark 2006, 156–157)

7   A patient undergoes computerized static perimetry. A certain area of the visual field in 1 eye fails to respond to the brightest stimulus available on the machine. What is this defect known as?

a. absolute scotoma
b. relative scotoma
c. baring of the blind spot
d. false positive response

ANSWER   **a.** absolute scotoma

EXPLANATION   A *scotoma* is an area within the contours of the visual field where vision is reduced. In perimetry, failure to respond to the largest, brightest stimulus that a machine can produce is known as an *absolute scotoma* (figure). (Newmark 2006, 158)

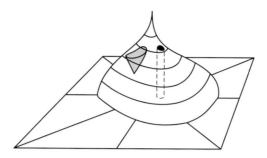

Defects in the island of vision. A deep scotoma (left), and an absolute scotoma that represents the normal blind spot (right). (Reproduced, with permission, from Newmark E, ed. *Ophthalmic Medical Assisting: An Independent Study Course,* 4th ed. San Francisco: American Academy of Ophthalmology; 2006.)

8   Which of the following Goldmann stimuli would outline the largest isopter in a human eye?

    a. I_{4e}
    b. II_{4e}
    c. III_{4e}
    d. V_{4e}

ANSWER   **d.** V_{4e}

EXPLANATION   Goldmann stimuli are labeled according to size with roman numerals, and intensity with subscripts. In this example, the intensities are all the same, only the size varies. The V_{4e} target is the largest and brightest intensity and easiest to see, therefore delineating the largest isopter. (Newmark 2006, 160)

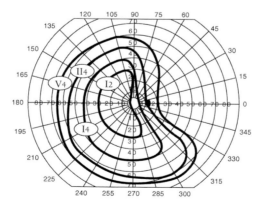

This Goldmann visual field chart is delineated by four stimuli with V_4 creating the largest isopter. It depicts a steep temporal defect of the right eye. (Reproduced, with permission, from Newmark E, ed. *Ophthalmic Medical Assisting: An Independent Study Course,* 4th ed. San Francisco: American Academy of Ophthalmology; 2006.)

9   What do the decibel numbers appearing on a visual field printout indicate?

    a. how loud the machine was during the stimulus presentations
    b. the actual location of the test points relative to fixation
    c. how much the maximum available stimulus intensity had been dimmed to still elicit a response from the patient

d. how much the minimum available stimulus intensity had been turned up to elicit a response from the patient

ANSWER   **c.** how much the maximum available stimulus intensity had been dimmed to still elicit a response from the patient

EXPLANATION   The decibel (dB) scale is a mathematical expression. It represents the placement of the dimming filters in front of the brightest test object available on a given machine. The dB numbers on the graph (figure) are a measure of the patient's ability to see dim stimuli. The higher the dB number, the dimmer the test object is, indicating relatively good sensitivity. (Newmark 2006, 161)

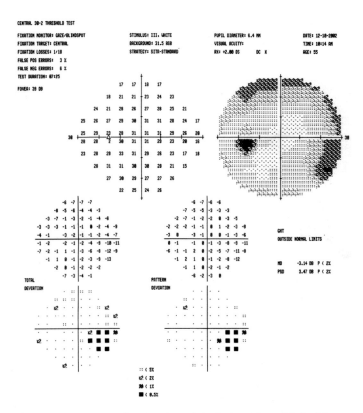

A computer-generated grayscale and decibel-numbered (left of the grayscale) rendering of a visual field as measured by static threshold perimetry. (Reproduced, with permission, from Newmark E, ed. *Ophthalmic Medical Assisting: An Independent Study Course,* 4th ed. San Francisco: American Academy of Ophthalmology; 2006.)

10   What is the name of the visual field test that isolates the blue cone?

a. white-on-white perimetry
b. kinetic perimetry
c. short wavelength automated perimetry
d. frequency-doubling perimetry

ANSWER   **c.** short wavelength automated perimetry

EXPLANATION   Short wavelength automated perimetry (SWAP) is a specific test that isolates the blue cone by using a blue stimulus on a yellow background. It can detect optic nerve damage 5 years before the standard test. White-on-white perimetry does not isolate the blue cone and is the standard visual field that is used in studying glaucoma and other conditions that cause visual field defects like an optic neuropathy or stroke. Kinetic perimetry uses a type of perimeter that employs a moving target. The frequency-doubling test (FDT) is another type of perimeter and is mainly used for glaucoma as a screening test employing a shimmering black-and-white stimulus. (Newmark 2006, 162)

11   A person with a bitemporal hemianopia is most likely to have what condition?

    a. pituitary tumor
    b. glaucoma
    c. occipital brain tumor
    d. cerebrovascular accident (stroke)

ANSWER   **a.** pituitary tumor

EXPLANATION   A pituitary tumor can compress the optic chiasm from below (figure), knocking out the nasal fibers from each eye that cross to the opposite side in the chiasm. This results in temporal visual field loss in each eye. Glaucoma causes defects that respect the horizontal midline. Brain tumors or strokes located posterior to the chiasm cause hemianopic defects on the opposite side. (Newmark 2006, 166, 168)

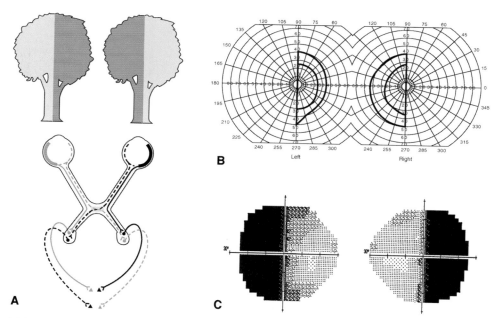

A bitemporal hemianopia due to a lesion (gray rectangle) of the optic chiasm. (A) The lesion has destroyed chiasmal crossing fibers from the nasal retinas (dotted lines). As a result, objects in the temporal half of the visual space (gray part of the tree) are not seen. (B) A Goldmann visual field chart of a bitemporal hemianopia. (C) A static chart of a similar defect. (Reproduced, with permission, from Newmark E, ed. *Ophthalmic Medical Assisting: An Independent Study Course,* 4th ed. San Francisco: American Academy of Ophthalmology; 2006.)

12   What is the most likely cause of a defect seen on a visual field that respects (does not cross) the vertical midline?

a. glaucoma
b. diabetic retinopathy
c. retinal scar
d. stroke

ANSWER   **d.** stroke

EXPLANATION   A vertical midline field defect is called a *homonymous hemianopia* (defects of the right [figure] or left half of the visual field in both eyes) and is caused by a stroke or brain tumor. In glaucoma, patients have a defect that respects the horizontal midline. The effect of diabetes on the retina can lead to visual impairment that can occur anywhere in the visual field. Scars will cause specific localized defects and do not respect the vertical or horizontal midline. (Newmark 2006, 166, 167)

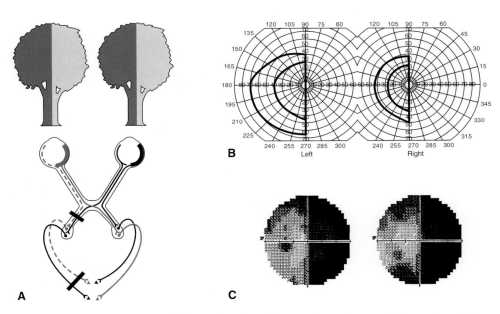

A right homonymous hemianopic defect resulting from a lesion in the optic tract or in the optic radiation of the visual cortex. (A) The lesion (black rectangles) has destroyed fibers of the optic tract or optic radiation from the temporal retina of the left eye (dotted line) and the nasal retina of the right eye (solid line). As a result, objects in the right half of the visual space (gray part of the tree) are not seen. (B) A Goldmann visual field chart of a right homonymous hemianopia. (C) A static chart of a right homonymous hemianopia. (Reproduced, with permission, from Newmark E, ed. *Ophthalmic Medical Assisting: An Independent Study Course,* 4th ed. San Francisco: American Academy of Ophthalmology; 2006)

13   What kind of defect does damage to the macula typically produce?

a. arcuate scotoma
b. Bjerrum scotoma
c. nasal step
d. central scotoma

ANSWER   **d.** central scotoma

EXPLANATION   The macula transmits information into the center of the visual field and therefore damage here would produce a central scotoma. Arcuate scotomas are often from vascular occlusions as the vessels in the eye take on an arc-shaped pattern. Patients with glaucoma often get arcuate scotomas, as there is cell loss along the nerve fiber layer in an arcuate pattern. A Bjerrum scotoma (a visual field defect starting at or near the physiologic blind spot and spreading nasally as a gradually widening band) is most often seen in glaucoma as well as a nasal step (the type of visual defect that appears as a step-like loss of vision at the outer nasal limit of the visual field). (Newmark 2006, 167)

14   In the visual fields shown, the condition depicted is most likely due to what cause?

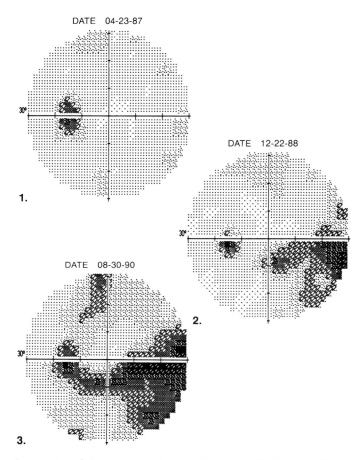

Progression of glaucomatous damage. The 3 visual fields shown illustrate the development and advancement of a visual field defect. Between the first and second visual fields, the patient developed a significant inferior nasal step. The third visual field illustrates the extension of this defect to the blind spot, as well as the development of a superior visual field loss (Humphrey 30–2 program). (Reproduced, with permission, from Cioffi GA, *Basic and Clinical Science Course,* Section 10: Glaucoma, American Academy of Ophthalmology, 2008–2009.)

a. macular degeneration
b. cataract
c. pituitary tumor
d. glaucoma

ANSWER   d. glaucoma

EXPLANATION   Glaucoma typically causes defects in the nasal visual field. The series of visual fields show worsening or progression, which is a hallmark of glaucoma. Macular degeneration would cause a defect in the center visual field. Cataract may cause a dimness of the entire visual field, but would not cause a localized defect, and a pituitary tumor would cause a temporal visual field defect in each eye. (Newmark 2006, 167)

15   What does daily calibration of a perimeter ensure?

    a. that patients will have similar test results each time
    b. that room lighting is consistent
    c. that the instrument has a consistent standard of sensitivity from day to day
    d. that the perimeter's computer works each day

ANSWER   **c.** that the instrument has a consistent standard of sensitivity from day to day

EXPLANATION   Calibration checks the perimeter's stimulus and background light intensities against a known standard and adjusts them as necessary to ensure that they remain the same each day. Calibration does not ensure that the room lighting is at the right level of brightness (it should be dark). Calibration does not provide a comprehensive test of the automated perimeter's computer. Calibration should be performed daily on nonautomated perimeters as well. Patients will vary in how they perform each day, even when the perimeter is precisely calibrated. (Newmark 2006, 169)

16   Which patient-related factors may improve the quality of a perimetry examination?

    a. removing the chinrest
    b. crying child in another room
    c. use of an automated perimeter
    d. presence of a perimetrist

ANSWER   **d.** presence of a perimetrist

EXPLANATION   The presence of a perimetrist (visual field examiner) allows the patient to concentrate on the examination, comfortable in the knowledge that he or she is being monitored and can ask for help. Also, a perimetrist can observe factors that may inhibit the patient's concentration, such as a chair adjusted too low or a crying baby in the distance. Patients with concentration difficulties often perform better on nonautomated perimeters. They tend to become drowsy or lose concentration during automated perimetry. (Newmark 2006, 168–171)

17   What can be said of the all-white visual field result shown in the figure?

    a. It is acceptable, and the test does not need to be repeated.
    b. It indicates that the patient is not paying attention and not pushing the response button.

c. It indicates that the patient does not understand the test and is constantly pushing the response button.

d. It indicates possible glaucoma damage.

ANSWER   c. It indicates that the patient does not understand the test and is constantly pushing the response button.

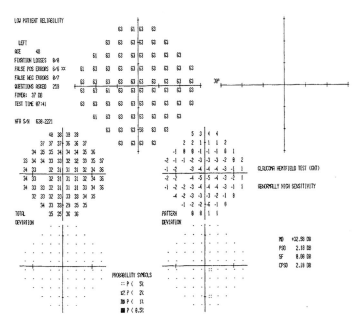

Visual field with 100% false positive responses. (Photo courtesy Neil T. Choplin, MD)

EXPLANATION   The figure shows 100% false positive responses. High false-positive rates indicate responses when no stimulus has been presented. A completely white field such as this offers no diagnostic information. It can result only from inappropriate pushing of the response button. (Newmark 2006, 170)

18   What factor affects the success of visual field testing?

a. asking the patient to look at the fixation point

b. asking the patient to follow the lights as they move

c. moving the test object 4° per second

d. keeping the room cold to help the patient stay awake

ANSWER   a. asking the patient to look at the fixation point

EXPLANATION   The effectiveness of the test is based on the patient's ability to maintain fixation at the fixation point. If the patient's eyes follow the lights, the central vision only is being tested. The usual suggested speed of movement of the test object in kinetic perimetry is 2° per second, or slower if the patient's reaction time is slow, as may be the case with elderly patients. A room should be a comfortable temperature, not too hot or cold—the patient could become sleepy in a hot room and uncomfortable in a cold room. (Newmark 2006, 171)

19   Two visual field tests from the same eye are performed sequentially on the same day. What is a possible explanation for the apparent improvement in the visual fields shown in the figure?

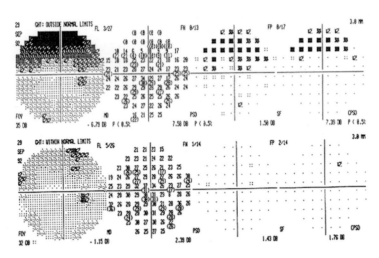

Two visual fields from the same eye performed sequentially on the same day. (Courtesy Neil T. Choplin, MD)

   a. The patient underwent a glaucoma procedure.
   b. The test was restarted after reinstructing the patient.
   c. The appropriate correcting lens was placed for the second test.
   d. The patient's upper eyelid was taped, correcting a ptosis.

ANSWER   **d.** The patient's upper eyelid was taped, correcting a ptosis.

EXPLANATION   The first visual field is a classic eyelid scotoma caused by ptosis. The other choices do not explain the apparent improvement on repeat testing during the same session. (Newmark 2006, 171)

20   Ptosis can affect what area of the visual field?

   a. superior
   b. inferior
   c. nasal
   d. temporal

ANSWER   **a.** superior

EXPLANATION   Ptosis is an abnormality in which the upper eyelid droops, cutting off the upper portion of the visual field. Holding up the eyelid with tape establishes a more accurate picture of the superior visual field. In glaucoma, the nasal visual field is usually the earliest area of visual field loss. Inferior visual field loss may be due to a superior retinal detachment. A temporal loss of field in both eyes is due to a lesion in the optic chiasm. (Newmark 2006, 171)

21   Two visual field tests from the same eye are performed sequentially on different days. In the figure, the result on the left was performed first. What is a possible explanation for the apparent improvement in the visual fields shown?

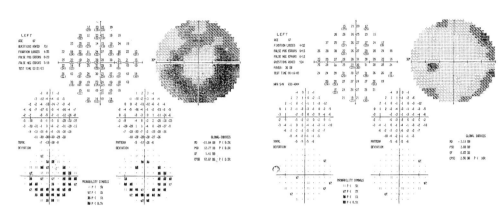

Two visual fields from the same eye performed sequentially on different days (the one on the left was performed first). (Courtesy Neil T. Choplin, MD)

a. The patient underwent a glaucoma procedure.
b. The patient was squinting during the first test.
c. The correcting lens was placed in the proper position for the second test.
d. The patient's upper eyelid was taped, correcting a ptosis.

ANSWER   c. The correcting lens was placed in the proper position for the second test.

EXPLANATION   The first field shows a correcting lens artifact, resulting from incorrect placement of the lens. The repeat field, with the lens in the correct position, eliminates the artifact. If the defect were real, lowering intraocular pressure would not result in this sort of improvement. Squinting and ptosis would not create such an artifact. (Newmark 2006, 171)

22   Which of the following is **not** a specialized visual field test?
a. SWAP
b. Ishihara plates
c. frequency doubling technology
d. tangent screen

ANSWER   b. Ishihara plates

EXPLANATION   Ishihara plates (pseudoisochromatic color plates) are used to test color vision (figure). Short wavelength automated perimetry (SWAP), frequency doubling technology (FDT), and tangent screen are all visual field tests. (Newmark 2006, 153–171)

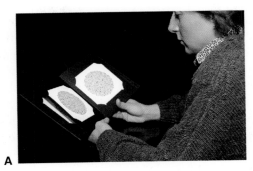

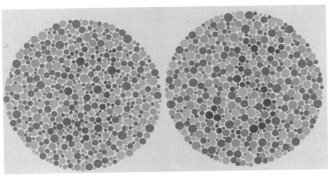

Pseudoisochromatic color plates used to test color vision. (A) The patient must detect numbers or figures embedded in an array of colored dots. (B) Pseudoisochromatic color plates in greater detail. (Part A reproduced, with permission, from Newmark E, ed. *Ophthalmic Medical Assisting: An Independent Study Course,* 4th ed. San Francisco: American Academy of Ophthalmology; 2006. Part B reproduced, with permission, from Regillo C, *Basic and Clinical Science Course*, Section 12: Retina and Vitreous. San Francisco: American Academy of Ophthalmology; 2004.)

23   All **except** which of the following are methods for testing the visual field?

a. Amsler grid
b. confrontation
c. refractometry
d. computerized static perimetry

ANSWER   c. refractometry

EXPLANATION   *Refractometry* refers to defining a patient's eyeglass prescription. This is a multifaceted measurement of refractive errors with a variety of specific instruments and techniques. The other methods are used for testing all or part of the visual field. (Newmark 2006, 63, 125–127, 161)

24   What is the most likely cause of a bitemporal visual field defect?

a. tumor near the chiasm
b. occipital lobe stroke
c. tumor near the optic radiations
d. aneurysm in the parietal lobe

ANSWER   a. tumor near the chiasm

EXPLANATION   Bitemporal defects are mostly from compression of the optic chiasm, where the two optic nerves merge at a point behind the eyes (figure). A tumor of the pituitary gland is the most likely cause. An occipital stroke causes a homonymous hemianopia as would an aneurysm in the parietal lobe or a tumor in the optic radiations, the nerve cells that travel to the right and left halves of the visual cortex at the back of the brain. Because 51% of the nerve fibers cross in the chiasm, a tumor or aneurysm occurring on one side of the brain causes a homonymous defect. Conditions in front of the chiasm cause visual defects in 1 eye. (Newmark 2006, 166, 168)

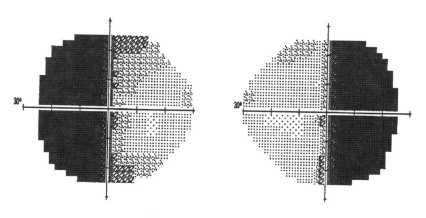

A bitemporal hemianopia, as seen on a computerized static visual field, due to a lesion of the optic chiasm. (Reproduced, with permission, from Newmark E, ed. *Ophthalmic Medical Assisting: An Independent Study Course,* 4th ed. San Francisco: American Academy of Ophthalmology; 2006.)

19 | SURGICAL ASSISTING IN ASC OR HOSPITAL-BASED OR

1   Which laser is used to cut a hole in a cloudy posterior capsule after cataract surgery?

 a. excimer
 b. krypton
 c. carbon dioxide
 d. Nd:YAG

ANSWER   d. Nd:YAG

EXPLANATION   When surgeons treat posterior capsule opacities they use a neodymium:yttrium-aluminum-garnet (Nd:YAG) laser. They may also use the Nd:YAG laser to cut a hole in the periphery of the iris to make an outflow channel for aqueous in patients with narrow-angle glaucoma. The excimer laser is used in corneal refractive surgery to remove a microscopic layer of corneal tissue. The krypton laser is used to photocoagulate retinal tissue for various conditions. It achieves greater photocoagulation through hazy media than argon lasers because of its longer wavelength. A carbon dioxide laser can be used during cosmetic surgery. It is typically used for laser resurfacing. It removes the superficial damaged layers of skin and irritates the underlying skin to stimulate new collagen. (Newmark 2006, 296; Yanoff 2008, 268)

2 When should the surgical site be first identified?

    a. when the patient signs the consent form
    b. when the patient is brought to the operating room
    c. after the final surgical scrub is performed
    d. after a timeout is called just prior to the start of the surgery

ANSWER   **a.** when the patient signs the consent form

EXPLANATION   Identifying the correct eye for surgery is an important preoperative step that should be repeated at each step listed above. However, it is important to first determine the surgical site, as soon as the patient gives consent and signs the consent forms to have the procedure. (Newmark 2006, 244)

3 Of the following, which suture material does the body break down?

    a. silk
    b. Mersilene
    c. polyglactin 910 (Vicryl)
    d. nylon

ANSWER   **c.** polyglactin 910 (Vicryl)

EXPLANATION   Polyglactin 910 (trade name Vicryl) is an example of an absorbable synthetic suture material. Absorbable natural suture material includes surgical gut and collagen. Permanent sutures that remain in place until removed include silk, nylon, polypropylene, or polyester fibers like Dacron and Mersilene. (Newmark 2006, 246)

4 Of the sutures listed, which one is the largest diameter?

    a. 10–0
    b. 8–0
    c. 4–0
    d. 6–0

ANSWER   **c.** 4–0

EXPLANATION   The 4–0 is the largest diameter of the sutures listed. With suture labeling, the higher the number, the smaller the diameter. (Newmark 2006, 246)

5 What medication is used prior to laser iridotomy?

    a. latanoprost
    b. glycerin
    c. timolol
    d. pilocarpine

ANSWER   **d.** pilocarpine

EXPLANATION   Pilocarpine is a miotic that is used to constrict the pupil prior to laser iridotomy. A constricted pupil increases the effectiveness of the laser procedure. Latanoprost is a prostaglandin analog used to treat glaucoma. A solution of glycerin for oral use is employed to lower acute elevations of IOP. Timolol is a beta-blocker used to treat glaucoma. (Newmark 2006, 85)

6   Regarding nonrefractive laser therapy, which phrase is accurate?

    a. is performed only by retinal specialists
    b. cannot be used to treat glaucoma
    c. requires preparing a sterile field
    d. is noninvasive

ANSWER   **d.** is noninvasive

EXPLANATION   Nonrefractive laser therapy is considered noninvasive because the tissues of the eye during the procedure are not exposed to any outside source of microorganisms. Therefore, a sterile field is not required. Frequently employed by retinal specialists, nonrefractive laser therapy is also used for glaucoma treatment and post-cataract capsulotomies (making an opening in a nontransparent posterior capsule after cataract surgery). (Newmark 2006, 296–297)

7   Which laser is used to treat proliferative diabetic retinopathy?

    a. argon
    b. excimer
    c. Nd:YAG
    d. confocal

ANSWER   **a.** argon

EXPLANATION   When surgeons treat proliferative diabetic retinopathy, they typically use an argon laser. They use the argon laser to create multiple burns in the retina to decrease the adverse effects. The argon laser may also be used to seal potential holes or tears, as well as treat chronic open-angle glaucoma by applying laser treatment to the trabecular meshwork. The excimer laser is used in corneal refractive surgery to remove a microscopic layer of corneal tissue. The Nd:YAG (neodymium:yttrium-aluminum-garnet) laser is used to open a cloudy posterior capsule after cataract surgery and also to create a hole in the peripheral iris to treat narrow angle glaucoma. Confocal laser scanning microscopy is a technique for obtaining high-quality optical images. (Newmark 2006, 296; Shetlar 2008)

8   Laser safety includes all **except** which of the following guidelines?

    a. Always wear approved protective eye goggles when assisting the ophthalmologist.
    b. Never attempt to demonstrate how the laser works without the correct knowledge, permission, and supervision.

    c. Be sure to perform laser maintenance by yourself at appropriate dates.

    d. Review the instruction manual for specific safeguards before assisting in the laser work area.

ANSWER   **c.** Be sure to perform laser maintenance by yourself at appropriate dates.

EXPLANATION   Lasers are powerful instruments that can cause damage if improperly tuned. It is important to allow only qualified service technicians to service lasers. Also, be sure to review the instruction manual for any specifics. (Newmark 2006, 297)

9   Common types of ophthalmic lasers include all **except** which of the following?

    a. argon

    b. excimer

    c. Nd:YAG

    d. fluorescein

ANSWER   **d.** fluorescein

EXPLANATION   Argon, excimer, and Nd:YAG (neodymium:yttrium-aluminum-garnet) lasers are all used as ophthalmic lasers. Fluorescein is dye with fluorescent properties that can be used to highlight degenerated corneal and conjunctival cells on the surface of the eye. This dye can also be used to highlight defects in the retinal structures and blood vessels when administered as an intravenous injection. (Newmark 2006, 296)

10   Steps to clean and protect surgical instruments after a procedure include all **except** which of the following?

    a. Remove all blood and tissues from disposable sharps before placing them in special sharps containers.

    b. Wear protective gloves.

    c. Cover delicate sharp instrument tips to reduce bends and misalignment and protect personnel.

    d. Count all sharps such as sutures, needles, and disposable blades to ensure none were left near the patient.

ANSWER   **a.** Remove all blood and tissues from disposable sharps before placing them in special sharps containers.

EXPLANATION   At no time should office personnel or waste collectors take the risk of cleaning disposable sharps. At the end of the case, disposable sharps should be placed directly into a specially marked sharps container. (Newmark 2006, 257–258)

11   During a chalazion surgery, the ophthalmic medical assistant's duties may include all **except** which of the following?

    a. holding the clamp during the incision and curettage

    b. using a cellulose sponge to blot any blood

c. passing a scalpel with the sharp end pointed toward the surgeon

d. anticipating the surgeon's needs during the procedure

ANSWER   **c.** passing a scalpel with the sharp end pointed toward the surgeon

EXPLANATION   The ophthalmic medical assistant should never pass surgical instruments with the sharp end pointed toward the surgeon. However, it can helpful if the medical assistant anticipates the surgeon's needs by holding the clamp or using a cellulose sponge to blot any blood. (Newmark 2006, 257)

Certified Ophthalmic Assistant Exam Study Guide

Self-Assessment Answer Key

Use this answer key to score the answers you recorded on the Self-Assessment Answer Sheet in the back of Section One.

Category 1:
History Taking

HIST 1   a
HIST 2   c
HIST 3   a
HIST 4   b
HIST 5   c
HIST 6   b
HIST 7   b
HIST 8   c

Category 2:
Pupillary Assessment

PA 1   a
PA 2   b
PA 3   a
PA 4   d
PA 5   a
PA 6   d
PA 7   a
PA 8   a
PA 9   d
PA 10   b

Category 3: Equipment Maintenance and Repair

MAIN 1   d
MAIN 2   c
MAIN 3   a
MAIN 4   b
MAIN 5   a
MAIN 6   d
MAIN 7   a
MAIN 8   d
MAIN 9   b
MAIN 10   b
MAIN 11   a
MAIN 12   d
MAIN 13   a
MAIN 14   d
MAIN 15   d
MAIN 16   c

MAIN 17   d
MAIN 18   b
MAIN 19   b
MAIN 20   c

Category 4: Lensometry

LENS 1   b
LENS 2   b
LENS 3   c
LENS 4   b
LENS 5   b
LENS 6   a
LENS 7   b
LENS 8   c
LENS 9   c
LENS 10   d
LENS 11   d
LENS 12   c

Category 5: Keratometry

KERA 1   d
KERA 2   b
KERA 3   a
KERA 4   b
KERA 5   c
KERA 6   c
KERA 7   a
KERA 8   c
KERA 9   b
KERA 10   d

Category 6: Medical Ethics, Legal, and Regulatory Issues

ETHS 1   b
ETHS 2   a
ETHS 3   c
ETHS 4   a
ETHS 5   c
ETHS 6   b
ETHS 7   d
ETHS 8   b

ETHS 9   d
ETHS 10   a
ETHS 11   a
ETHS 12   b
ETHS 13   b
ETHS 14   d
ETHS 15   a
ETHS 16   c
ETHS 17   d
ETHS 18   c
ETHS 19   a
ETHS 20   d
ETHS 21   b

Category 7:
Microbiology

MICRO 1   b
MICRO 2   d
MICRO 3   b
MICRO 4   a
MICRO 5   c
MICRO 6   a

Category 8:
Pharmacology

PHAR 1   d
PHAR 2   d
PHAR 3   a
PHAR 4   b
PHAR 5   b
PHAR 6   c
PHAR 7   c
PHAR 8   a
PHAR 9   a
PHAR 10   a
PHAR 11   a
PHAR 12   b
PHAR 13   a
PHAR 14   a
PHAR 15   b
PHAR 16   d
PHAR 17   c
PHAR 18   a

PHAR 19   c
PHAR 20   b
PHAR 21   d
PHAR 22   c
PHAR 23   b
PHAR 24   a
PHAR 25   a
PHAR 26   b
PHAR 27   d
PHAR 28   d
PHAR 29   a
PHAR 30   b
PHAR 31   c
PHAR 32   c

Category 9:
Ocular Motility

MOTI 1   a
MOTI 2   a
MOTI 3   d
MOTI 4   a
MOTI 5   a
MOTI 6   c

Category 10: In-Office Minor Surgical Procedures

SURG 1   b
SURG 2   a
SURG 3   d
SURG 4   c
SURG 5   d
SURG 6   b
SURG 7   d
SURG 8   d
SURG 9   b
SURG 10   c
SURG 11   d
SURG 12   d
SURG 13   c
SURG 14   d
SURG 15   a
SURG 16   d

Category 11:
Ophthalmic Patient
Services and Education

PAT 1   d
PAT 2   d
PAT 3   d
PAT 4   d
PAT 5   a
PAT 6   d
PAT 7   c
PAT 8   c
PAT 9   a
PAT 10   d
PAT 11   d
PAT 12   b
PAT 13   c
PAT 14   a
PAT 15   a
PAT 16   d
PAT 17   c
PAT 18   c
PAT 19   a
PAT 20   c
PAT 21   c
PAT 22   d
PAT 23   a
PAT 24   d
PAT 25   a
PAT 26   c
PAT 27   b
PAT 28   c
PAT 29   b
PAT 30   c
PAT 31   c
PAT 32   a
PAT 33   c
PAT 34   a
PAT 35   b
PAT 36   a
PAT 37   a
PAT 38   c
PAT 39   c
PAT 40   a
PAT 41   c
PAT 42   a
PAT 43   a
PAT 44   c
PAT 45   b
PAT 46   a
PAT 47   d
PAT 48   c
PAT 49   b
PAT 50   c
PAT 51   c
PAT 52   d
PAT 53   a

PAT 54   a
PAT 55   c
PAT 56   d
PAT 57   b
PAT 58   d
PAT 59   c
PAT 60   a
PAT 61   a

Category 12:
Ophthalmic Imaging

IMAG 1   a
IMAG 2   c
IMAG 3   a
IMAG 4   d
IMAG 5   b
IMAG 6   a
IMAG 7   b
IMAG 8   b
IMAG 9   d
IMAG 10   b
IMAG 11   a
IMAG 12   a
IMAG 13   d
IMAG 14   c
IMAG 15   c
IMAG 16   d
IMAG 17   b
IMAG 18   c
IMAG 19   d
IMAG 20   b
IMAG 21   a
IMAG 22   c

Category 13:
Refractometry

REF 1   c
REF 2   b
REF 3   d
REF 4   c
REF 5   a
REF 6   c
REF 7   c
REF 8   c
REF 9   b
REF 10   b
REF 11   d
REF 12   c
REF 13   d
REF 14   b

Category 14:
Spectacle Skills

SPEC 1   a
SPEC 2   c

SPEC 3   c
SPEC 4   c
SPEC 5   a
SPEC 6   d
SPEC 7   a
SPEC 8   b
SPEC 9   d
SPEC 10   b
SPEC 11   c
SPEC 12   c
SPEC 13   b
SPEC 14   b

Category 15:
Supplemental Skills

SUPP 1   a
SUPP 2   c
SUPP 3   c
SUPP 4   b
SUPP 5   b
SUPP 6   a
SUPP 7   c
SUPP 8   a
SUPP 9   d
SUPP 10   b
SUPP 11   a
SUPP 12   c
SUPP 13   b
SUPP 14   d
SUPP 15   a
SUPP 16   d
SUPP 17   b

Category 16:
Tonometry

TON 1   b
TON 2   c
TON 3   a
TON 4   c
TON 5   b
TON 6   c
TON 7   c
TON 8   c
TON 9   d
TON 10   a
TON 11   a
TON 12   c
TON 13   d

Category 17:
Visual Assessment

VA 1   b
VA 2   d
VA 3   c
VA 4   c

VA 5   a
VA 6   d
VA 7   d
VA 8   b
VA 9   a
VA 10   b
VA 11   c
VA 12   a
VA 13   c
VA 14   c
VA 15   c
VA 16   c

Category 18:
Visual Fields

VF 1   b
VF 2   d
VF 3   d
VF 4   d
VF 5   a
VF 6   a
VF 7   a
VF 8   d
VF 9   c
VF 10   c
VF 11   a
VF 12   d
VF 13   d
VF 14   d
VF 15   c
VF 16   d
VF 17   c
VF 18   a
VF 19   d
VF 20   a
VF 21   c
VF 22   b
VF 23   c
VF 24   a

Category 19: Surgical
Assisting in ASC or
Hospital-Based OR

ASST 1   d
ASST 2   a
ASST 3   c
ASST 4   c
ASST 5   d
ASST 6   d
ASST 7   a
ASST 8   c
ASST 9   d
ASST 10   a
ASST 11   c

Practice Test

1　How does the examiner determine if a patient has abnormal tear-film breakup?

    a. Look for corneal and conjunctival staining with rose bengal dye.

    b. Place strips of filter paper in the lower fornix of each eye for 5 minutes.

    c. Stain with fluorescein and check the tear meniscus height.

    d. Stain the tears with fluorescein, ask the patient not to blink, and record when blue patches appear.

2　What does pachymetry measure?

    a. corneal thickness

    b. axial length of the globe (eyeball)

    c. intraocular pressure

    d. corneal curvature

3　Which statement is correct regarding the Schirmer test performed with topical anesthetic?

    a. It measures reflex tear production.

    b. It measures basal tear production.

    c. It measures both basal and reflex tear production.

    d. It is poorly tolerated by patients.

4　Generally, the history starts with the chief complaint. It can be defined as which of the following?

    a. the interviewer's troubles with co-workers

    b. the main reason for the patient's visit to the doctor

    c. less important goals for the doctor-patient interaction

    d. what hurts the patient most, at the present time

5　When asking about a patient's symptoms, which of the following questions is most important?

    a. When did the symptoms begin?

    b. Who were you with when the symptoms went away?

    c. Who brought you here today?

    d. Did you do anything to deserve this?

6   Why is the recording of the patient's medication important at every visit?

    a. Medications rarely have ocular side effects.
    b. Patients' medications frequently change.
    c. Patients take their medications exactly as prescribed.
    d. The doctor already remembers what the patient takes.

7   What is the first step in testing pupillary response?

    a. Ask the patient to focus on a distant target.
    b. Turn the room lights off and on.
    c. Shine the light on one pupil while observing the response of the other pupil.
    d. Dilate with only phenylephrine before testing.

8   The pupillary exam is most important in the diagnosis of what condition?

    a. conjunctivitis
    b. cataract
    c. optic nerve disease
    d. amblyopia

9   Which approach is an acceptable method of disinfecting an applanation tonometer prism?

    a. Soak it for 5 minutes in acetone.
    b. Soak it for 5 minutes in standard household bleach.
    c. Soak it for 5 minutes in hydrogen peroxide 3%.
    d. Soak it for 5 minutes in sterile water.

10   The slit-lamp biomicroscope requires what kind of special attention?

    a. Use a soft facial tissue to clean the mirrored surfaces.
    b. Roll the machine back and forth to loosen any sticky movements.
    c. Turn off the machine when not in use.
    d. Change the bulb with a bulb that has the same base.

11   What statement best applies to the lasers in the office?

    a. Office personnel are responsible for cleaning and maintaining the laser.
    b. Laser use requires approved protective eyewear for the assistant.
    c. The laser can be demonstrated to the patient prior to the procedure.
    d. They use little energy.

12   What statement applies to calibration of the manual keratometer?

    a. Check calibration periodically using a blank lens.
    b. Check calibration periodically using a known lens power.
    c. Check calibration periodically using metal spheres of known curvature.
    d. Perform calibration if it seems out of alignment.

13 What is the purpose of keratometry?

   a. to measure the power of the lens of the eye
   b. to help determine the maximum visual field
   c. to measure the eyeglass prescription
   d. to measure the corneal curvature

14 To obtain an accurate measurement in keratometry, where should the reticule be placed?

   a. in the center of the bottom-right circle
   b. outside the upper-right circle
   c. in the center of the left circle
   d. inside the upper-right circle

15 A keratometry reading of 43.00 is entered into an intraocular lens (IOL) calculation as 45.00. What error will result?

   a. approximately 3 D of change in postoperative refractive error
   b. approximately 2 D of change in postoperative refractive error
   c. approximately 1 D of change in postoperative refractive error
   d. no significant error in postoperative refractive error

16 Which of the following best describes a requirement for becoming a certified ophthalmic assistant (COA)?

   a. Complete formal training by physically attending coursework sessions.
   b. Obtain a sponsoring optician's signature.
   c. Pass a written examination.
   d. Complete the COA workbook.

17 Which one of these is considered a HIPAA violation?

   a. discussing a patient's condition in the elevator
   b. discussing a patient's condition with the patient
   c. discussing a patient's condition with another health provider that takes care of the same patient
   d. discussing the patient's condition with one of their family members with their permission

18 Prior to examination by the physician, a patient tells the assistant that he has been taking illegal drugs. Which of the following documentation procedures is most appropriate for the ophthalmic medical assistant?

   a. Document the conversation in the medical record.
   b. Highlight this finding for attention by the physician.
   c. Write this information on a separate paper for physician review.
   d. Do not document compromising details unless relevant to the ocular condition.

19   Which of the following methods achieves sterilization?

   a. autoclaving

   b. wiping with 1:100 bleach solution

   c. freezing

   d. wiping with 70% alcohol

20   Coding is dynamic, and standards change over time. A basic distinction can be made between codes for diagnoses and codes for procedures and services. What is the coding system to classify surgical procedures?

   a. E codes

   b. V codes

   c. CPT codes

   d. ICD-9-CM codes

21   Which of the following is required for proper aseptic technique?

   a. protecting an article's sterility before and during use

   b. always wearing sterile gloves

   c. sterilizing disposable items before reuse

   d. refrigerating sterile eyedrops after opening

22   Which statement is correct regarding ocular infections?

   a. Ocular involvement is rarely seen in patients infected with human immunodeficiency virus.

   b. Herpes simplex virus infections can be recurrent despite treatment.

   c. Herpes simplex virus rarely causes blindness in the United States.

   d. Gram-positive bacteria cause ocular infections, but Gram-negative bacteria do not.

23   Which of the following is an advantage of ointments, compared to eyedrops?

   a. less blurred vision

   b. less burning

   c. longer contact with the eye

   d. washes away easily

24   Before a mydriatic drug is used, which of the following should be checked in the patient?

   a. corneal sensitivity

   b. color vision

   c. ocular motility

   d. depth of the anterior chamber angle

25   Which of the following actions can the patient perform to reduce systemic absorption of a topically administered medication?

    a. Blink frequently.
    b. Apply light pressure at the inner corner of the eyelids.
    c. Squeeze the eyelids together.
    d. Use more than 1 drop of medication.

26   The use of cycloplegic agents is contraindicated in patients with which condition?

    a. open-angle glaucoma
    b. inflammatory glaucoma
    c. narrow-angle glaucoma
    d. congenital glaucoma

27   What problem can long-term treatment of topical anesthetics create?

    a. toxicity to the corneal endothelium
    b. bacterial overgrowth
    c. glaucoma
    d. delayed healing

28   Natamycin, amphotericin, and ketoconazole are medications used to treat what type of infections?

    a. fungal infections
    b. bacterial infections
    c. viral infections
    d. parasitic infections

29   Which statement is correct regarding prescription medications?

    a. Many prescriptions may be called in to the pharmacy by the ophthalmic medical assistant.
    b. All prescriptions must include the doctor's license number.
    c. Prescriptions to be filled as needed must be undated.
    d. Only controlled substances such as narcotics require refill instructions.

30   Which one of the following items must the ophthalmic medical assistant know the location of in case of an acute allergic reaction?

    a. injectable epinephrine
    b. acetaminophen
    c. aspirin
    d. timolol

31   What condition results in the eyes shifting involuntarily in a rhythmic motion?

    a. strabismus
    b. amblyopia
    c. nystagmus
    d. circles of eccentricity

32   *Eso deviation* refers to an ocular malalignment. In what direction would this eye deviate?

    a. out
    b. up
    c. down
    d. in

33   Which of the following is most representative of comitant strabismus?

    a. a nerve paralysis causing 1 or more muscles to function abnormally
    b. muscle scarring, as in Graves disease
    c. a deviation that measures the same amount in all fields of gaze
    d. a deviation that varies in different fields of gaze

34   The principal reason to perform a cover-uncover test is to determine or assess which of the following?

    a. ocular alignment
    b. fusion
    c. stereopsis
    d. amblyopia

35   On Worth 4-dot testing, a patient sees 3 dots. What does this probably represent?

    a. fusion
    b. suppression
    c. diplopia
    d. stereopsis

36   Which of the following is the responsibility of the ophthalmic medical assistant?

    a. ensuring sterility of the surgical area and materials
    b. holding the instrument tray
    c. allowing the surgeon to open and organize all equipment and supplies
    d. answering patient questions about the specifics of the surgery and expected outcome

37   Which of the following statements applies to absorbable sutures used in ophthalmic surgery?

    a. They must be removed after 2 weeks.
    b. They are composed of nylon.

c. They will dissolve over time.
d. They are composed of Dacron.

38   What instrument is used to inject saline into the lacrimal sac?

a. punctal dilator
b. clamp
c. cannula
d. probes

39   What is the most common and serious complication of an intravitreal injection?

a. cataract
b. intravitreal hemorrhage
c. endophthalmitis
d. retinal detachment

40   Which of the following applies during minor ophthalmic surgery?

a. The ophthalmic medical assistant helps to provide better operative exposure for the surgeon.
b. Only disposable instruments and materials are used.
c. Protective attire is required only for the surgeon.
d. Draping is not necessary.

41   Which extraocular muscle adducts the eye (turns it inward)?

a. superior rectus
b. inferior oblique
c. lateral rectus
d. medial rectus

42   What tissues comprise the uveal tract?

a. iris, crystalline lens, retina
b. choroid, ciliary body, crystalline lens
c. ciliary body, crystalline lens, retina
d. iris, ciliary body, choroid

43   What layer of corneal tissue pumps fluid out of the cornea?

a. Bowman's membrane
b. stroma
c. Descemet's membrane
d. endothelium

44   Herpes zoster ("shingles") often affects the ophthalmic branch of the trigeminal nerve. This condition, called *herpes zoster ophthalmicus*, is caused by a flare-up of which viral condition?

   a. measles
   b. mumps
   c. chicken pox
   d. rubella

45   Why is it important to ask questions about a family history of eye disease?

   a. Some ocular diseases are hereditary.
   b. Curiosity is a natural human trait.
   c. Patients may volunteer that they were adopted.
   d. Their in-laws may have a genetic disease.

46   A young child has lost an eye as a result of trauma. Which of the following recommendations would be most appropriate for this patient?

   a. The patient should wear a black patch so people will know of the disability.
   b. The patient should not participate in contact sports.
   c. The patient should wear polycarbonate spectacle lenses.
   d. The patient should be referred for psychological counseling.

47   Which of the following patients belongs at the top of the triage list?

   a. a patient with eye itching for 1 week
   b. a patient who noted a red spot on the white part of the eye this morning
   c. a patient referred for cataract surgery by an optometrist who sends many patients
   d. a patient who complains of new floaters with flashing lights

48   Which statement is correct regarding physically disabled patients?

   a. Wheelchair wheels must remain unlocked when moving the patient to the exam chair.
   b. Patient mobility may be compromised by strokes, arthritis, multiple sclerosis, and other conditions.
   c. Patients in wheelchairs should always be accompanied.
   d. Driver's license vision standards apply to operators of motorized wheelchairs (scooters).

49   Which of the following systemic symptoms is most typical for a patient with new-onset diabetes mellitus?

   a. increased thirst and urination
   b. a rapid heart rate and nervousness
   c. numbness and tingling in the extremities
   d. pain in the temple and jaw

50 What is the function of a pressure patch?

a. prevents eyelid movement
b. ensures bilateral eyelid closure
c. prevents movement of the globe
d. prevents rupture of the globe

51 Which pair of eye muscle's action is to elevate the globe?

a. superior rectus and superior oblique
b. superior oblique and inferior oblique
c. superior rectus and inferior oblique
d. superior rectus and lateral rectus

52 Which lens treatment, tint, or coating provides the most effective reduction in glare from sunlight reflecting from bodies of water?

a. photochromatic lenses
b. polarized lenses
c. antireflective coatings
d. neutral density filters

53 Which of the following is **not** a medical reason to apply a pressure patch?

a. to limit bleeding after a surgical wound
b. to cover a "black eye"
c. to limit bacteria from reaching the eye
d. to immobilize the eyelids to promote corneal epithelial healing

54 What is the first step in using a manual lensmeter to determine the power of an eyeglass lens?

a. Correctly position the eyeglasses in the lensmeter.
b. Turn the power drum to a high minus position.
c. Turn the power drum to a high plus position.
d. Focus the eyepiece of the lensmeter.

55 What change must be made on the lensmeter to be able to read a cylinder lens that is in the plus convention into the minus format?

a. Change the axis 180°.
b. Change the axis 45°.
c. Change the axis 90°.
d. Change the axis to zero.

56 The following occurs while taking a lensmeter reading: the single lines focus at −2.50; the triple lines focus at −1.00 with the axis at 085°. What would be the eyeglass prescription?

    a. −2.50 −1.00 axis 175
    b. −2.50 +1.50 axis 085
    c. −1.00 −2.50 axis 175
    d. −3.50 −1.00 axis 085

57 What is the best test to document the shape and average number of corneal endothelial cells in a patient with Fuchs corneal dystrophy?

    a. fundus photography
    b. external photography
    c. slit-lamp photography
    d. specular microscopy photography

58 When an ophthalmologist orders a photographic test to document the position of the eyelid in a patient with ptosis, what type of ophthalmic photography is indicated?

    a. fundus photography
    b. external photography
    c. slit-lamp photography
    d. specular microscopy photography

59 The figure shows an example of what type of ophthalmic test?

    a. specular microscopy
    b. slit-lamp photography
    c. fundus photography
    d. slit-lamp gonioscopic photography

60 What ophthalmic photographic test uses the techniques of sclerotic scatter and retroillumination to evaluate the cornea and media opacities?

    a. fundus photography
    b. external photography
    c. slit-lamp photography
    d. specular microscopy photography

61 How do optical coherence tomography (OCT), GDx scanning laser polarimetry with variable corneal compensation, and the Heidelberg retinal tomograph allow the ophthalmologist to interpret the 3-dimensional depiction of the optic nerve and retinal nerve fiber layer in glaucoma patients?

    a. by comparison with a database of age-matched "normal" patients
    b. by comparison with a database of other patients with glaucoma
    c. by comparison with a database of other age-matched patients with glaucoma
    d. by comparison with a database of "normal" patients

62   What test is used to measure the axial length of the globe in preparation for intraocular lens calculations for patients about to undergo cataract surgery?

    a. B-scan (B-mode) ultrasonography
    b. 3-dimensional ultrasonography
    c. A-scan (A-mode) ultrasonography
    d. optical coherence tomography

63   Patients with what type of allergy should not undergo intravenous indocyanine green (ICG) fundus angiography?

    a. peanuts
    b. penicillin
    c. morphine
    d. shellfish

64   What is the focal length of a spectacle lens with a power of +5.00 diopters?

    a. 0.50 meters
    b. 5.00 meters
    c. 2.00 meters
    d. 0.20 meters

65   What type of lens best corrects hyperopia with astigmatism?

    a. prism
    b. cylindrical lens
    c. spherical lens
    d. spherocylindrical lens

66   If a ray of light traveling through a lens is deviated 1 centimeter at 1 meter of distance, what is the power of the lens?

    a. 1 diopter of myopia
    b. 1 diopter of astigmatism
    c. 1 prism diopter
    d. 1 diopter of add

67   During retinoscopy, what type of light reflex is seen in a myopic eye?

    a. moves in the same direction as the streak of light
    b. moves in the opposite direction as the streak of light
    c. does not appear to have any movement
    d. streak of light has a red glow

68   An automated objective refractor is helpful in what tasks?

    a. making an estimate of the prescription for eyeglasses
    b. refining a subjective refraction

c. determining the refractive error in a patient with moderate cataracts

d. measuring the refractive error in a patient with very small pupils

69   A cross cylinder may be used to refine the refractive error correction of eyes with what condition?

   a. diplopia
   b. astigmatism
   c. presbyopia
   d. hypermetropia

70   In tightening or replacing a screw on an eyeglass frame, a droplet of what substance should be used to secure the screw?

   a. epoxy resin
   b. white glue
   c. shellac
   d. clear fingernail polish

71   How can light transmission through an eyeglass lens be increased?

   a. applying an antireflective coating onto the lens
   b. tinting the lens a light yellow color
   c. increasing the size of the lens
   d. placing a high polish on both the front and back surfaces of the lens

72   What is the base curve of an eyeglass lens?

   a. the curve on the front surface of the lens
   b. the curve on the back surface of the lens
   c. the smaller of the front and back surface curves
   d. the larger of the front and back surface curves

73   What is the size of the area applanated on the cornea by the Goldmann tonometer?

   a. 1 square millimeter
   b. 3.06 square millimeters
   c. 10 square millimeters
   d. irrelevant to the measurement

74   What statement applies to a patient with an intraocular pressure reading of 25 mm Hg on Goldmann applanation tonometry?

   a. definitely has glaucoma
   b. definitely does not have glaucoma
   c. may actually have lower intraocular pressure
   d. should be rechecked 1 hour later

75 The tip of the Goldmann tonometer is round, yet the mires seen during applanation tonometry appear as 2 semicircles. How is this achieved?

  a. the use of a prism within the tip
  b. the optics of the cornea itself
  c. the use of a high plus lens
  d. an artifact of a circular object touching the cornea

76 Which of the following methods might be the most accurate for measuring intraocular pressure in an eye with a scarred, irregular cornea?

  a. Goldmann tonometry
  b. palpation
  c. air-puff tonometry
  d. Tono-Pen

77 Of the following, what is the accurate second part of the phrase, "The higher the scale reading on the Schiøtz tonometer … "?

  a. the higher the intraocular pressure
  b. the lower the intraocular pressure
  c. the less the cornea has been indented
  d. the more resistance to compression

78 What is the derivation of the word *laser*?

  a. light amplified by sensory emission of radiation
  b. light amplification by stimulated emission of radiation
  c. light amplitude synonymous with emitted radiation
  d. longitudinal aberrations of seismographic emitted radio waves

79 Which phrase applies to aseptic technique?

  a. is usually not necessary in an office procedure
  b. limited to sterilizing instruments and wearing gloves
  c. is important because it reduces the risk of infection
  d. is only required in a hospital

80 The ophthalmic medical assistant's duties related to surgery include which of the following?

  a. getting the patient's consent
  b. sterilizing the instruments
  c. filling out the encounter form
  d. talking to the patient's family

81 What is the most common opacity affecting the ocular media?

    a. cataract
    b. vitreous hemorrhage
    c. glaucoma
    d. scotoma

82 If the patient cannot see the big "E" (20/400) on the Snellen acuity chart when best corrected, what does this indicate?

    a. The patient is blind.
    b. The patient should have cataract surgery.
    c. The patient should be tested for count fingers (CF), hand motions (HM), or light perception (LP) vision.
    d. The patient has a constricted visual field.

83 Which phrase applies to the super pinhole test?

    a. measures current vision after a refraction
    b. requires a dilated pupil
    c. can be performed regardless of the capability of the patient
    d. is rarely helpful

84 Which statement is correct regarding visual acuity testing in the pediatric patient?

    a. Visual acuity cannot be assessed for the preliterate child.
    b. A papoose board is routinely used for infants.
    c. The examination method is not different than for adults.
    d. A principle goal is to assess visual acuity without intimidating the child.

85 What does the pinhole acuity test measure?

    a. the patient's corrected vision with a proper refraction
    b. the best vision the patient would be expected to achieve if the media were clear
    c. the patient's ability to read
    d. the patient's vision with both eyes looking through pinholes

86 Visual potential tests include which of the following?

    a. testing for near vision
    b. refracting the patient after dilation
    c. PAM, interferometer, and super pinhole
    d. visual field

87 A patient complains of transient shimmering vision that affected the right half of the visual field in each eye. The shimmering vision lasted about 20 minutes and resolved completely. The diagnosis is ophthalmic migraine (migraine without the headache). Which part of the brain was affected by the transient blood vessel spasm?

a. the right occipital area
b. the left occipital area
c. the right frontal cortex
d. the left frontal cortex

88   Where anatomically do the optic nerve fibers come together and reorganize?

a. optical center
b. optic chiasm
c. fovea
d. visual pathway

89   The Humphrey computerized perimeter is an automated system for measuring a patient's visual field. How are test points presented?

a. kinetic strategy
b. static testing
c. contrast sensitivity
d. object size differences

90   What is the term for an abnormal visual field that is missing the right or left quadrant?

a. Bjerrum scotoma
b. hemianopia
c. quadrantanopia
d. normal visual field

91   When performing a visual field test, if the pupil is smaller than 2 mm, what should you do?

a. Continue with the test.
b. Request permission to dilate the pupil.
c. Use a more powerful lens.
d. Perform the visual field test twice.

92   During perimetry, what is the usual reason for taping the upper eyelid to keep it out of the field of view?

a. provides a break for restless patients
b. increases the amount of light captured by the eye
c. improves the test results if the patient has astigmatism
d. improves the test results if the patient has ptosis

93   An elderly patient with no past eye or medical problems presents with nausea, sudden onset of right eye pain, and blurred vision with haloes around lights. What is the likely explanation?

    a. mature cataract
    b. corneal ulcer
    c. endophthalmitis
    d. acute angle-closure glaucoma

94   What function does the Farnsworth-Munsell D-15 test have in office practice?

    a. tests color vision
    b. measures central retinal thickness
    c. measures corneal curvature
    d. tests distance visual acuity

95   Glare testing is most useful in the evaluation of which of the following?

    a. cataract
    b. glaucoma
    c. macular degeneration
    d. uveitis

96   If the axial length of the eye measured is shorter than the actual axial length, how will the postoperative refraction be affected?

    a. no effect
    b. more hyperopia than anticipated
    c. more myopia than anticipated
    d. more astigmatism than anticipated

97   A patient has an axial length of 26.00 mm and K readings of 44.00 D. Which of the following statements is true?

    a. This is average, and the patient will have no significant refractive error.
    b. This is a short eye with flat curvature, and the patient will be hyperopic.
    c. This is a long eye with flat curvature, and the patient will be myopic.
    d. This is a long eye with steep curvature, and the patient will be myopic.

98   Evaluation of color vision is often performed using which of the following?

    a. direct ophthalmoscope
    b. pseudoisochromatic test plates
    c. Schirmer test
    d. Worth four-dot test

99   A patient has increased corneal thickness. What problem may arise when this patient's intraocular pressure (IOP) is measured with an applanation tonometer?

    a. A higher concentration of anesthetic is necessary to numb the cornea.
    b. The mires (prism image) will be distorted and irregular.
    c. The IOP reading will be falsely low.
    d. The IOP reading will be falsely high.

100   If the anterior chamber is shallow, the flashlight test will show which of the following?

    a. The iris is evenly illuminated.
    b. The iris is shadowed on the temporal side.
    c. The iris is shadowed on the nasal side.
    d. The pupil is unable to constrict normally.

Certified Ophthalmic Assistant Exam Study Guide

Practice Test Answer Sheet

Record your responses to the questions in Section Three on this answer sheet. Use the *Practice Test Answer Key* at the back of Section Four to score your work.

1 _____	26 _____	51 _____	76 _____
2 _____	27 _____	52 _____	77 _____
3 _____	28 _____	53 _____	78 _____
4 _____	29 _____	54 _____	79 _____
5 _____	30 _____	55 _____	80 _____
6 _____	31 _____	56 _____	81 _____
7 _____	32 _____	57 _____	82 _____
8 _____	33 _____	58 _____	83 _____
9 _____	34 _____	59 _____	84 _____
10 _____	35 _____	60 _____	85 _____
11 _____	36 _____	61 _____	86 _____
12 _____	37 _____	62 _____	87 _____
13 _____	38 _____	63 _____	88 _____
14 _____	39 _____	64 _____	89 _____
15 _____	40 _____	65 _____	90 _____
16 _____	41 _____	66 _____	91 _____
17 _____	42 _____	67 _____	92 _____
18 _____	43 _____	68 _____	93 _____
19 _____	44 _____	69 _____	94 _____
20 _____	45 _____	70 _____	95 _____
21 _____	46 _____	71 _____	96 _____
22 _____	47 _____	72 _____	97 _____
23 _____	48 _____	73 _____	98 _____
24 _____	49 _____	74 _____	99 _____
25 _____	50 _____	75 _____	100 _____

Practice Test Answers and Explanations

1   How does the examiner determine if a patient has abnormal tear-film breakup?

    a. Look for corneal and conjunctival staining with rose bengal dye.

    b. Place strips of filter paper in the lower fornix of each eye for 5 minutes.

    c. Stain with fluorescein and check the tear meniscus height.

    d. Stain the tears with fluorescein, ask the patient not to blink, and record when blue patches appear.

ANSWER   **d.** Stain the tears with fluorescein, ask the patient not to blink, and record when blue patches appear.

EXPLANATION   All items listed are related to tests preformed in evaluating dry eye patients. Rose bengal dye stains "sick cells" on the cornea and conjunctiva. Option "b" describes a Schirmer tear test. The tear meniscus height is the amount of tears along the lower eyelid margin against the eyeball.

Tear-film breakup time (TBUT) is measured by staining the tear film with fluorescein and observing through the slit-lamp biomicroscope and cobalt blue light how many seconds it takes for breaks to occur in the tear film. The patient must hold the eyes open without blinking. The person conducting the test should not touch the eyelid during this time, as it changes the surface tension of the tear film. As the tear film breaks up, dark blue patches appear in the faint green tint of the fluorescein. (Patel 2003, 27)

2   What does pachymetry measure?

    a. corneal thickness

    b. axial length of the globe (eyeball)

    c. intraocular pressure

    d. corneal curvature

ANSWER   **a.** corneal thickness

EXPLANATION   Modern pachymeters use ultrasonography to measure corneal thickness. The axial length of the globe is measured with A-scan ultrasonography. Several different instruments measure intraocular pressure: applanation tonometer, Schiøtz tonometer, Tono-Pen (electronic) tonometer, noncontact tonometer. Corneal curvature is measured by keratometry or corneal topography. (Newmark 2006, 144)

3   Which statement is correct regarding the Schirmer test performed with topical anesthetic?

    a. It measures reflex tear production.
    b. It measures basal tear production.
    c. It measures both basal and reflex tear production.
    d. It is poorly tolerated by patients.

ANSWER   **b.** It measures basal tear production.

EXPLANATION   The Schirmer test (figure) measures tear output. The Schirmer I tear test is performed without topical anesthetic. It measures the production of both basal and reflex tears. Basal tear production makes up the corneal tear film, helping to maintain the visual clarity and comfort of the cornea. If the basal tear film is not adequate the corneal tear film begins to dry up and becomes uncomfortable, causing reflex tearing. Patients with dry eye syndrome frequently complain that they "tear all the time." This is the reflex tearing, which occurs in response to basal tear inadequacy. The Schirmer II tear test is performed with topical anesthetic. With anesthetic, only basal tears are measured. With anesthesia, the test is well tolerated by patients. (Newmark 2006, 135)

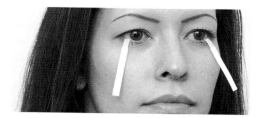

The Schirmer test, in which the amount of wetting of the paper strips is a measure of tear flow. (Reproduced, with permission, from Newmark E, *Ophthalmic Medical Assisting: An Independent Study Course*, 4th ed. San Francisco: American Academy of Ophthalmology; 2006.)

4   Generally, the history starts with the chief complaint. It can be defined as which of the following?

    a. the interviewer's troubles with co-workers
    b. the main reason for the patient's visit to the doctor
    c. less important goals for the doctor-patient interaction
    d. what hurts the patient most, at the present time

ANSWER   **b.** the main reason for the patient's visit to the doctor

EXPLANATION   The chief complaint is the main reason for the patient's visit, usually in the patient's own words and placed in quotes. The problems of the interviewer, while important, are not the focus of the ophthalmic and medical history. Patients may have secondary goals for the visit, which should be noted in the chart, but the chief complaint is the single most important reason for the visit, which may or may not involve discomfort. (Newmark 2006, 114, 281)

5   When asking about a patient's symptoms, which of the following questions is most important?

    a. When did the symptoms begin?
    b. Who were you with when the symptoms went away?

    c. Who brought you here today?

    d. Did you do anything to deserve this?

ANSWER   **a.** When did the symptoms begin?

EXPLANATION   The onset of the symptom is important, as is its frequency, intensity, severity, location, modifiers (what makes it better or worse?) and its attribution (what does the patient think is causing it?). Learning the answers to all of these questions would be important to fully understand the symptom, but who the patient was with when the symptom went way and who brought the patient to the office are far less important. Asking the patient a question like "Did you do anything to deserve this?" is value-laden and inappropriate. (Newmark 2006, 113–116)

6   Why is the recording of the patient's medication important at every visit?

    a. Medications rarely have ocular side effects.

    b. Patients' medications frequently change.

    c. Patients take their medications exactly as prescribed.

    d. The doctor already remembers what the patient takes.

ANSWER   **b.** Patients' medications frequently change.

EXPLANATION   Patients frequently change their medications, and it is for this reason their medications should be reviewed and recorded at every visit. It is not true that patients always take their medicines as prescribed or that doctors always remember what medicines their patients take. Finally, medications frequently have ocular side effects. (Newmark 2006, 116)

7   What is the first step in testing pupillary response?

    a. Ask the patient to focus on a distant target.

    b. Turn the room lights off and on.

    c. Shine the light on one pupil while observing the response of the other pupil.

    d. Dilate with only phenylephrine before testing.

ANSWER   **a.** Ask the patient to focus on a distant target.

EXPLANATION   By having the patient focus on a distant target, you control changes in pupil size from accommodation, which allows you to see a stable pupil size for measurement and to stimulate that pupil with light to see its reactions and the reactions of the fellow eye. Turning the room lights on and off is not the first step in pupillary testing. Pupil response of the fellow eye (consensual response) is an important part of pupillary testing, but not the first step. Pupils should never be dilated before pupillary testing. Phenylephrine is a weak pupillary dilator and should not be used in testing pupillary response. (Newmark 2006, 125–126)

8   The pupillary exam is most important in the diagnosis of what condition?

    a. conjunctivitis
    b. cataract
    c. optic nerve disease
    d. amblyopia

ANSWER   **c.** optic nerve disease

EXPLANATION   The only condition listed in which an abnormality of pupillary function might be expected is optic nerve disease. Without an afferent pupillary defect, the diagnosis of unilateral optic nerve disease is unlikely. Conjunctivitis is an inflammation of the conjunctiva. Cataract is a cloudiness of the crystalline lens. Amblyopia is poor vision due to visual deprivation in early childhood. (Trobe 2006:11)

9   Which approach is an acceptable method of disinfecting an applanation tonometer prism?

    a. Soak it for 5 minutes in acetone.
    b. Soak it for 5 minutes in standard household bleach.
    c. Soak it for 5 minutes in hydrogen peroxide 3%.
    d. Soak it for 5 minutes in sterile water.

ANSWER   **c.** Soak it for 5 minutes in hydrogen peroxide 3%.

EXPLANATION   Disinfection of the applanation tonometer prism can be accomplished by wiping the prism with an alcohol swab and letting it air dry. Another technique is to soak the prism for 5 minutes in hydrogen peroxide 3% or in 1 part household bleach to 9 parts water. Acetone degrades plastic, and its use is not approved for tonometer prism disinfection. Standard household bleach is too concentrated for soaking and must be diluted as noted above. Sterile water is not acceptable for disinfecting applanation tonometer prisms, but it is useful for rinsing the tips after disinfecting. (Newmark 2006, 294)

10   The slit-lamp biomicroscope requires what kind of special attention?

    a. Use a soft facial tissue to clean the mirrored surfaces.
    b. Roll the machine back and forth to loosen any sticky movements.
    c. Turn off the machine when not in use.
    d. Change the bulb with a bulb that has the same base.

ANSWER   **c.** Turn off the machine when not in use.

EXPLANATION   The mirror of the slit-lamp biomicroscope must be cleaned gently with a dust brush or nonabrasive, lint-free cloth, photographic lens cleaner, using downward strokes only. If the joystick of the machine become difficult to move, sewing machine oil can be used to lubricate the ball joint area after careful cleaning. All equipment (other than rechargers) should be turned off when not in use. Bulb replacement must follow approved guidelines and procedures and are more specific than having the same base. (Newmark 2006, 292)

11   What statement best applies to the lasers in the office?

    a. Office personnel are responsible for cleaning and maintaining the laser.
    b. Laser use requires approved protective eyewear for the assistant.
    c. The laser can be demonstrated to the patient prior to the procedure.
    d. They use little energy.

ANSWER   **b.** Laser use requires approved protective eyewear for the assistant.

EXPLANATION   Only qualified service technicians should maintain the lasers. Protective eyewear should be worn when assisting the ophthalmologist in the laser work area. Do not demonstrate how the laser works without proper permission, training, and supervision. Every laser is very powerful and used for specific purposes. (Newmark 2006, 297)

12   What statement applies to calibration of the manual keratometer?

    a. Check calibration periodically using a blank lens.
    b. Check calibration periodically using a known lens power.
    c. Check calibration periodically using metal spheres of known curvature.
    d. Perform calibration if it seems out of alignment.

ANSWER   **c.** Check calibration periodically using metal spheres of known curvature.

EXPLANATION   Calibration of the manual keratometer is checked periodically by using metal spheres of known curvature. Only a repair technician should repair the unit if it seems out of alignment. (Newmark 2006, 291)

13   What is the purpose of keratometry?

    a. to measure the power of the lens of the eye
    b. to help determine the maximum visual field
    c. to measure the eyeglass prescription
    d. to measure the corneal curvature

ANSWER   **d.** to measure the corneal curvature

EXPLANATION   A keratometer measures the corneal curvature. The power of the lens is not measured by this device. Visual fields are measured by various types of perimeters. The eyeglass prescription is based on many factors including the length of the eye, corneal curvature, and lens power, and not only corneal curvature. (Newmark 2006, 73)

14   To obtain an accurate measurement in keratometry, where should the reticule be placed?

    a. in the center of the bottom-right circle
    b. outside the upper-right circle
    c. in the center of the left circle
    d. inside the upper-right circle

ANSWER   **a.** in the center of the bottom-right circle

EXPLANATION   The reticule is placed in the bottom-right circle as a primary condition for accurate measurements. The other answers are incorrect and would not give accurate results. The keratometer was designed to have the reticule in the bottom-right circle as the standard for measurements. (Newmark 2006, 75)

15   A keratometry reading of 43.00 is entered into an intraocular lens (IOL) calculation as 45.00. What error will result?

    a. approximately 3 D of change in postoperative refractive error
    b. approximately 2 D of change in postoperative refractive error
    c. approximately 1 D of change in postoperative refractive error
    d. no significant error in postoperative refractive error

ANSWER   **b.** approximately 2 D of change in postoperative refractive error

EXPLANATION   A 45.00 D keratometry reading is 2 D steeper than the correct 43.00 D. The patient's eye would falsely indicate it is more myopic by 2 D and that error will reduce the IOL power calculation by 2 D. Consequently, the patient will have a postoperative hyperopic refractive error. Most patients want to have a minimal need for glasses after cataract surgery, and a miscalculation of the IOL power can result in an unhappy patient. (Newmark 2006, 120–121, 264)

16   Which of the following best describes a requirement for becoming a certified ophthalmic assistant (COA)?

    a. Complete formal training by physically attending coursework sessions.
    b. Obtain a sponsoring optician's signature.
    c. Pass a written examination.
    d. Complete the COA workbook.

ANSWER   **c.** Pass a written examination.

EXPLANATION   To become a certified ophthalmic assistant, one must successfully pass the JCAHPO comprehensive examination. Formal training is not required to sit for the examination, and the sponsor must be an ophthalmologist, not an optician. Although study guides like the one you are using now help you prepare for the exam, there is no additional workbook required for COA certification. (JCAHPO 2009 [see Suggested Reading]; Newmark 2006, 4)

17   Which one of these is considered a HIPAA violation?

   a. discussing a patient's condition in the elevator
   b. discussing a patient's condition with the patient
   c. discussing a patient's condition with another health provider that takes care of the same patient
   d. discussing the patient's condition with one of their family members with their permission

ANSWER   **a.** discussing a patient's condition in the elevator

EXPLANATION   The patient's condition should never be discussed in common areas where other people can overhear the comments. (Newmark 2006, 7, 228)

18   Prior to examination by the physician, a patient tells the assistant that he has been taking illegal drugs. Which of the following documentation procedures is most appropriate for the ophthalmic medical assistant?

   a. Document the conversation in the medical record.
   b. Highlight this finding for attention by the physician.
   c. Write this information on a separate paper for physician review.
   d. Do not document compromising details unless relevant to the ocular condition.

ANSWER   **c.** Write this information on a separate paper for physician review.

EXPLANATION   The medical chart is a legal record, and the physician is responsible for its accuracy. Therefore, information that you believe could compromise the patient or others (eg, abuse, sexual practices, or illegal drug taking) should best be assessed by the supervising ophthalmologist to determine whether, and if so how, it should be included in the medical record. Medical judgment may be necessary. Policy may vary by individual practice. One approach is to write this information down on a separate paper for physician review or discuss it with the physician prior to incorporating it into the medical record. (Newmark 2006, 117)

19   Which of the following methods achieves sterilization?

   a. autoclaving
   b. wiping with 1:100 bleach solution
   c. freezing
   d. wiping with 70% alcohol

ANSWER   **a.** autoclaving

EXPLANATION   Of the methods mentioned, only autoclaving (which uses steam under pressure to kill microorganisms and spores) can achieve sterilization. Wiping with antiseptic solutions of 1:100 bleach or 70% alcohol will reduce microbial contamination. Freezing is often used in laboratories to preserve and store viruses and bacteria. (Newmark 2006, 104)

20   Coding is dynamic, and standards change over time. A basic distinction can be made between codes for diagnoses and codes for procedures and services. What is the coding system to classify surgical procedures?

a. E codes
b. V codes
c. CPT codes
d. ICD-9-CM codes

ANSWER   c. CPT codes

EXPLANATION   Current Procedural Terminology (CPT) codes are used for evaluation and treatments including surgical procedures. International Classification of Diseases, ninth revision, clinical modification (ICD-9-CM) and the supplementary codes V and E are used to describe the patient's diagnosis and other modifying factors. (Newmark 2006, 278–279)

21   Which of the following is required for proper aseptic technique?

a. protecting an article's sterility before and during use
b. always wearing sterile gloves
c. sterilizing disposable items before reuse
d. refrigerating sterile eyedrops after opening

ANSWER   a. protecting an article's sterility before and during use

EXPLANATION   The sterility of an instrument or container needs to be maintained before and during its use. Sterilized instruments may be handled only on a part that will not come in contact with the patient or with other nonsterile materials. Sterile gloves need not be used as long as sterile instruments are not handled at the functional surface of the article. Disposable items are to be discarded after a single use and not re-sterilized. Sterility of eyedrops is maintained by chemical preservatives and preventing physical contamination of the bottle tip and cap. Refrigeration is not required. (Newmark 2006, 105–106)

22   Which statement is correct regarding ocular infections?

a. Ocular involvement is rarely seen in patients infected with human immunodeficiency virus.
b. Herpes simplex virus infections can be recurrent despite treatment.
c. Herpes simplex virus rarely causes blindness in the United States.
d. Gram-positive bacteria cause ocular infections, but Gram-negative bacteria do not.

ANSWER   b. Herpes simplex virus infections can be recurrent despite treatment.

EXPLANATION   Despite effective treatments, herpes simplex virus (HSV) infections continue to be one of the leading causes of blindness in the United States. This is due to the high recurrence rate of HSV infections. Ocular infection with cytomegalovirus is commonly seen in patients infected with human immunodeficiency virus (HIV). Both Gram-positive and Gram-negative bacteria cause ocular infections. (Newmark 2006, 98)

23   Which of the following is an advantage of ointments, compared to eyedrops?

    a. less blurred vision
    b. less burning
    c. longer contact with the eye
    d. washes away easily

ANSWER   **c.** longer contact with the eye

EXPLANATION   Ointments tend to cause more blurring of vision and are more difficult to wash away. They can equally cause burning as eyedrops. The major advantage of ointments is that they have longer contact time with the eye. (Newmark 2006, 80)

24   Before a mydriatic drug is used, which of the following should be checked in the patient?

    a. corneal sensitivity
    b. color vision
    c. ocular motility
    d. depth of the anterior chamber angle

ANSWER   **d.** depth of the anterior chamber angle

EXPLANATION   Mydriatics dilate the pupil. This can precipitate an attack of angle-closure glaucoma in patients with narrow anterior chamber angles by crowding the angle with iris tissue as the pupil enlarges. The corneal sensitivity test should be checked before anesthetic drops are applied. For best results, color vision and ocular motility should be checked before dilation, but an enlarged pupil does not appreciably affect the result of the test. (Newmark 2006, 81)

25   Which of the following actions can the patient perform to reduce systemic absorption of a topically administered medication?

    a. Blink frequently.
    b. Apply light pressure at the inner corner of the eyelids.
    c. Squeeze the eyelids together.
    d. Use more than 1 drop of medication.

ANSWER   **b.** Apply light pressure at the inner corner of the eyelids.

EXPLANATION   Applying light pressure at the inner corner of the eyelids limits the amount of drug that drains into the nasolacrimal system. An alternate method is gently closing the eyelids for 2 minutes without blinking. The other choices actually increase systemic absorption by causing more medication to drain out through the nasolacrimal system. (Newmark 2006, 82)

26   The use of cycloplegic agents is contraindicated in patients with which condition?

a. open-angle glaucoma
b. inflammatory glaucoma
c. narrow-angle glaucoma
d. congenital glaucoma

ANSWER   c. narrow-angle glaucoma

EXPLANATION   Cycloplegics such as tropicamide can precipitate an attack of acute angle-closure glaucoma by crowding the iris tissue into the angle as the pupil enlarges. There is no contraindication in using cycloplegics in the other conditions. (Newmark 2006:83)

27   What problem can long-term treatment of topical anesthetics create?

a. toxicity to the corneal endothelium
b. bacterial overgrowth
c. glaucoma
d. delayed healing

ANSWER   d. delayed healing

EXPLANATION   Topical anesthetics, while good at decreasing corneal pain, may delay re-epithelization (resurfacing) of the corneal epithelium, increasing risk of corneal infection. They do not cause glaucoma or an overgrowth of bacteria. They do not penetrate deep into the corneal tissue to affect the endothelium. (Newmark 2006, 84)

28   Natamycin, amphotericin, and ketoconazole are medications used to treat what type of infections?

a. fungal infections
b. bacterial infections
c. viral infections
d. parasitic infections

ANSWER   a. fungal infections

EXPLANATION   Natamycin, amphotericin, and ketoconazole are antifungal agents. These should be used with a proven or highly suspicious diagnosis of fungal disease, as some may be toxic to the cornea. (Newmark 2006, 86)

29   Which statement is correct regarding prescription medications?

a. Many prescriptions may be called in to the pharmacy by the ophthalmic medical assistant.
b. All prescriptions must include the doctor's license number.
c. Prescriptions to be filled as needed must be undated.
d. Only controlled substances such as narcotics require refill instructions.

ANSWER   **a.** Many prescriptions may be called in to the pharmacy by the ophthalmic medical assistant.

EXPLANATION   Many prescriptions can be called in to the pharmacy; controlled substances such as narcotics are an exception. The doctor's medical license number is required only for controlled substances. All prescriptions should be dated. Authorization or lack of authorization for refills can be noted on all prescriptions. (Newmark 2006, 89)

30   Which one of the following items must the ophthalmic medical assistant know the location of in case of an acute allergic reaction?

   a. injectable epinephrine
   b. acetaminophen
   c. aspirin
   d. timolol

ANSWER   **a.** injectable epinephrine

EXPLANATION   Injectable epinephrine, as well as cortisone, diphenhydramine (Benadryl), oxygen, diazepam (Valium), smelling salts or spirits of ammonia all may be necessary in the treatment of an acute allergic reaction. Although it is helpful to have over-the-counter analgesics (acetaminophen and aspirin) available in the office, they ordinarily are not used in an acute allergic reaction. Timolol is used to lower intraocular pressure. (Newmark 2006, 90)

31   What condition results in the eyes shifting involuntarily in a rhythmic motion?

   a. strabismus
   b. amblyopia
   c. nystagmus
   d. circles of eccentricity

ANSWER   **c.** nystagmus

EXPLANATION   Nystagmus is the rhythmic shifting of the eyes in a side-to-side, up-and-down, or rotary motion. Strabismus is misalignment of the eyes. Amblyopia is decreased vision from early visual deprivation. Circles of eccentricity refers to the mapping of the visual field. (Newmark 2006, 31)

32   *Eso deviation* refers to an ocular malalignment. In what direction would this eye deviate?

   a. out
   b. up
   c. down
   d. in

ANSWER   **d.** in

EXPLANATION   The figure shows types of heterotropia. *Eso deviation* refers to an eye that turns inward. *Exo* refers to an outward turn, *hyper* refers to an upward turn, and *hypo* refers to a downward turn. (Bradford 2004,126–127; Newmark 2006, 31)

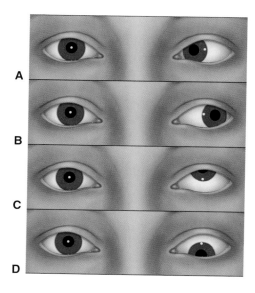

Types of heterotropia. Note the corneal light reflex. (A) Esotropia (inward). (B) Exotropia (outward). (C) Hypertropia (upward). (D) Hypotropia (downward). (Illustration by Christine Gralapp, CMI)

33   Which of the following is most representative of comitant strabismus?

a. a nerve paralysis causing 1 or more muscles to function abnormally
b. muscle scarring, as in Graves disease
c. a deviation that measures the same amount in all fields of gaze
d. a deviation that varies in different fields of gaze

ANSWER   c. a deviation that measures the same amount in all fields of gaze

EXPLANATION   *Comitant strabismus* refers to a constant deviation in all fields of gaze. Muscle scarring or nerve paralysis typically results in a deviation that is not constant in all fields of gaze (incomitant strabismus). (Newmark 2006, 31)

34   The principal reason to perform a cover-uncover test is to determine or assess which of the following?

a. ocular alignment
b. fusion
c. stereopsis
d. amblyopia

ANSWER   a. ocular alignment

EXPLANATION   The cover-uncover test determines ocular alignment. Fusion is measured by the Worth 4-dot test. Stereopsis is measured by the Titmus fly and circle test. Amblyopia is measured by visual acuity testing. (Newmark 2006, 123)

35   On Worth 4-dot testing, a patient sees 3 dots. What does this probably represent?

a. fusion
b. suppression
c. diplopia
d. stereopsis

ANSWER   b. suppression

EXPLANATION   The Worth 4-dot test (figure) is designed to determine how a patient uses his or her 2 eyes together. If a misalignment or other abnormality is interfering with fusion, the brain may ignore the image from 1 eye (suppression). A patient with suppression will see fewer than 4 dots. A patient with normal fusion will see 4 dots. A patient with diplopia will see more than 4 dots. Stereopsis is measured with the Titmus fly and circle test. (Newmark 2006, 123)

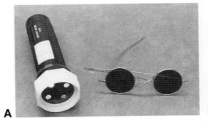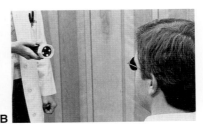

The Worth 4-dot test. (A) The flashlight target, which illuminates 4 dots: 2 green, 1 red, and 1 white. The eyeglasses are fitted with a red and a green filter. (B) The flashlight is held in front of the patient, who wears the colored eyeglasses. (Reproduced, with permission, from Newmark E, ed. *Ophthalmic Medical Assisting: An Independent Study Course*, 4th ed. San Francisco: American Academy of Ophthalmology, 2006.)

36   Which of the following is the responsibility of the ophthalmic medical assistant?

a. ensuring sterility of the surgical area and materials
b. holding the instrument tray
c. allowing the surgeon to open and organize all equipment and supplies
d. answering patient questions about the specifics of the surgery and expected outcome

ANSWER   a. ensuring sterility of the surgical area and materials

EXPLANATION   Surgical instruments are typically arranged on a sterile tray in order of expected use; instruments may be passed by the ophthalmic medical assistant to the surgeon. The assistant opens and prepares equipment and supplies to be used during the procedure. It is appropriate that the surgeon answer patient's questions about the specifics of the surgical procedure or its outcome. Assistants may answer questions about what to expect during the minor surgery visit, and what they may feel during and after the procedure. (Newmark 2006, 245, 257)

37   Which of the following statements applies to absorbable sutures used in ophthalmic surgery?

    a. They must be removed after 2 weeks.
    b. They are composed of nylon.
    c. They will dissolve over time.
    d. They are composed of Dacron.

ANSWER   **c.** They will dissolve over time.

EXPLANATION   Absorbable sutures degrade over time and do not need to be removed. The usual types of absorbable sutures include natural gut material or a synthetic suture material such as polyglactin 910 (brand name Vicryl). Nonabsorbable sutures are made of silk, nylon, polypropylene, or polyester fibers such as Dacron. They are intended to be permanent and are not removed. (Newmark 2006, 246)

38   What instrument is used to inject saline into the lacrimal sac?

    a. punctal dilator
    b. clamp
    c. cannula
    d. probes

ANSWER   **c.** cannula

EXPLANATION   A cannula is a hollow blunt-tipped, needle-like instrument that is ideal for testing the flow of tears through the nasolacrimal drainage system. After injection of saline through the punctum into the lacrimal sac, a partial or total lacrimal sac obstruction can be detected. If there is resistance to injection of the saline, leakage of saline out of either punctum or ballooning of the lacrimal sac may indicate obstruction. If the nasolacrimal system is patent (open), saline drains into the nose/throat quite easily. (Newmark 2006, 248)

39   What is the most common and serious complication of an intravitreal injection?

    a. cataract
    b. intravitreal hemorrhage
    c. endophthalmitis
    d. retinal detachment

ANSWER   **c.** endophthalmitis

EXPLANATION   An intravitreal injection involves placing medication into the vitreous. Endophthalmitis is the most common and potentially most serious risk of an intravitreal injection, although all of the options listed are possible. Some studies place the risk of endophthalmitis after an intravitreal injection at about the same incidence as that seen after intraocular surgery (<1%). (Newmark 2006, 253)

40   Which of the following applies during minor ophthalmic surgery?

a. The ophthalmic medical assistant helps to provide better operative exposure for the surgeon.
b. Only disposable instruments and materials are used.
c. Protective attire is required only for the surgeon.
d. Draping is not necessary.

ANSWER   a. The ophthalmic medical assistant helps to provide better operative exposure for the surgeon.

EXPLANATION   During surgery, the duties of the ophthalmic medical assistant center on providing better operative exposure for the surgeon. This might involve holding a clamp or using a cellulose sponge to blot away blood so the surgeon's view is unobstructed. Disposable instruments and materials are often used in ophthalmic surgery; other instruments are washed and rinsed before being sterilized for reuse. The surgeon and assistant both require appropriate protective attire. Draping preserves the sterility of the surgical field after the preoperative prepping is completed. (Newmark 2006, 255–257)

41   Which extraocular muscle adducts the eye (turns it inward)?

a. superior rectus
b. inferior oblique
c. lateral rectus
d. medial rectus

ANSWER   d. medial rectus

EXPLANATION   Adduction of the eye is the function of the medial rectus (figure). The lateral rectus abducts the eye (turns it outward). The superior rectus primarily elevates the eye, and the inferior oblique elevates, but also abducts, and extorts the eye. (Newmark 2006, 13–14)

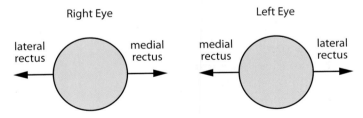

Lateral and medial rectus muscles of the eye.

42   What tissues comprise the uveal tract?

a. iris, crystalline lens, retina
b. choroid, ciliary body, crystalline lens
c. ciliary body, crystalline lens, retina
d. iris, ciliary body, choroid

ANSWER   **d.** iris, ciliary body, choroid

EXPLANATION   The iris, ciliary body, and choroid are pigmented vascular tissues that are contiguous within the eye (figure). The crystalline lens and retina are not part of the uveal tract. (Newmark 2006, 18–19)

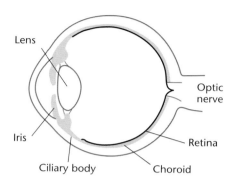

The uveal tract. The iris, ciliary body, and choroid in relation to other structures of the eye. (Reproduced, with permission, from Newmark E, ed. *Ophthalmic Medical Assisting: An Independent Study Course,* 4th ed. San Francisco: American Academy of Ophthalmology; 2006.)

43   What layer of corneal tissue pumps fluid out of the cornea?

   a. Bowman's membrane
   b. stroma
   c. Descemet's membrane
   d. endothelium

ANSWER   **d.** endothelium

EXPLANATION   The corneal endothelium pumps fluid out of the cornea whereby the cornea maintains a thickness and clarity important for visual function (figure). Bowman's membrane supports the corneal epithelium. The corneal stroma provides structural integrity to the cornea and Descemet's membrane supports the corneal endothelium. (Newmark 2006, 17)

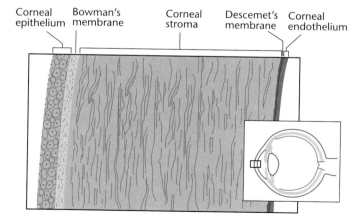

The five layers of the cornea. (Reproduced, with permission, from Newmark E, ed. *Ophthalmic Medical Assisting: An Independent Study Course,* 4th ed. San Francisco: American Academy of Ophthalmology; 2006.)

44   Herpes zoster ("shingles") often affects the ophthalmic branch of the trigeminal nerve. This condition, called *herpes zoster ophthalmicus*, is caused by a flare-up of which viral condition?

 a. measles
 b. mumps
 c. chicken pox
 d. rubella

ANSWER   c. chicken pox

EXPLANATION   Although infection with the chicken pox virus in childhood usually results in lifelong immunity, a few individuals with a weakening of their immune system will have a flare-up of the virus along a nerve root resulting in a herpes zoster infection ("shingles"). The eyelid, conjunctiva, cornea, and anterior chamber are usual sites for herpes zoster ocular involvement. Measles, mumps, and rubella are viral diseases that do not reactivate and cause an eye disease. (Newmark 2006, 49, 98)

45   Why is it important to ask questions about a family history of eye disease?

 a. Some ocular diseases are hereditary.
 b. Curiosity is a natural human trait.
 c. Patients may volunteer that they were adopted.
 d. Their in-laws may have a genetic disease.

ANSWER   a. Some ocular diseases are hereditary.

EXPLANATION   Asking questions about a family history of eye disease and medical disease is important because many conditions may be hereditary, including early-onset glaucoma. While curiosity may be natural, it is not the reason a complete medical history is important. The questions asked must be for the patient's best interests. The medical history of the patient's relatives by marriage is not as important for hereditary diseases because they are not related by blood. (Newmark 2006, 116)

46   A young child has lost an eye as a result of trauma. Which of the following recommendations would be most appropriate for this patient?

 a. The patient should wear a black patch so people will know of the disability.
 b. The patient should not participate in contact sports.
 c. The patient should wear polycarbonate spectacle lenses.
 d. The patient should be referred for psychological counseling.

ANSWER   c. The patient should wear polycarbonate spectacle lenses.

EXPLANATION   Polycarbonate lenses are impact-resistant and would better protect the noninjured eye from accidental trauma. A black patch would not protect the uninjured eye. With the proper protective eyewear, single-eyed patients can enjoy contact sports. Young children generally adjust to a disability without professional counseling. (Newmark 2006, 179)

47   Which of the following patients belongs at the top of the triage list?

    a. a patient with eye itching for 1 week
    b. a patient who noted a red spot on the white part of the eye this morning
    c. a patient referred for cataract surgery by an optometrist who sends many patients
    d. a patient who complains of new floaters with flashing lights

ANSWER   **d.** a patient who complains of new floaters with flashing lights

EXPLANATION   The concept of triage is to evaluate the patient with the most serious problem and for whom a delay might worsen the condition and eventual outcome. A patient with new floaters and flashing lights might have a new vitreous detachment and an associated retinal tear and should come in immediately and therefore be at the top of the triage list. A patient with itching eyes for 1 week may be bothered and should be evaluated, but the situation does not require immediate attention. The patient with a red spot on the conjunctiva probably has a subconjunctival hemorrhage and may need reassurance from an exam but does not have an emergency problem. A cataract referral does not represent an emergency. (Newmark 2006, 215–217)

48   Which statement is correct regarding physically disabled patients?

    a. Wheelchair wheels must remain unlocked when moving the patient to the exam chair.
    b. Patient mobility may be compromised by strokes, arthritis, multiple sclerosis, and other conditions.
    c. Patients in wheelchairs should always be accompanied.
    d. Driver's license vision standards apply to operators of motorized wheelchairs (scooters).

ANSWER   **b.** Patient mobility may be compromised by strokes, arthritis, multiple sclerosis, and other conditions.

EXPLANATION   A number of conditions can affect a patient's mobility, and ophthalmic medical assistants may expect to help physically disabled patients in wheelchairs during a visit. Wheelchair wheels must be locked and immobilized to allow safe patient transfer to the examination chair. Patients in wheelchairs/scooters may navigate safely without assistance or meeting driver's licensure visual standards. (Newmark 2006, 237)

49   Which of the following systemic symptoms is most typical for a patient with new-onset diabetes mellitus?

    a. increased thirst and urination
    b. a rapid heart rate and nervousness
    c. numbness and tingling in the extremities
    d. pain in the temple and jaw

ANSWER   **a.** increased thirst and urination

EXPLANATION   Elevated glucose levels often cause metabolic disturbances, resulting in increased thirst and urination. Hyperthyroidism may be associated with a fast heart rate and nervousness. Patients with multiple sclerosis may have numbness and tingling in their extremities. Giant cell arteritis may present with pain in the temple and jaw. (Newmark 2006, 238)

50   What is the function of a pressure patch?

    a. prevents eyelid movement
    b. ensures bilateral eyelid closure
    c. prevents movement of the globe
    d. prevents rupture of the globe

ANSWER   **a.** prevents eyelid movement

EXPLANATION   A pressure patch is used to prevent lid movement or limit bleeding. It is applied over the closed eyelid. The patch does not prevent globe movement, and it should never be applied to a ruptured globe. (Newmark 2006, 254)

51   Which pair of eye muscle's action is to elevate the globe?

    a. superior rectus and superior oblique
    b. superior oblique and inferior oblique
    c. superior rectus and inferior oblique
    d. superior rectus and lateral rectus

ANSWER   **c.** superior rectus and inferior oblique

EXPLANATION   The superior rectus and the inferior oblique are elevators of the eye. The superior oblique is an eye depressor. The lateral rectus is an abductor (turns the eye lateral or outward). (Newmark 2006, 13–14)

52   Which lens treatment, tint, or coating provides the most effective reduction in glare from sunlight reflecting from bodies of water?

    a. photochromatic lenses
    b. polarized lenses
    c. antireflective coatings
    d. neutral density filters

ANSWER   **b.** polarized lenses

EXPLANATION   Light that is reflected from horizontal surfaces such as bodies of water consists largely of polarized light. This means that the polarized lenses will effectively block most of the reflected light causing glare. Photochromatic lenses become darker in bright light but they and neutral density filters do not preferentially block reflected light or polarized light. However, both of these lenses reduce the overall amount of light entering the eye. Antireflective coatings reduce reflection from the lenses, thus increasing the amount of light transmitted to the eye, not reducing it. (Newmark 2006, 179–180)

53   Which of the following is **not** a medical reason to apply a pressure patch?

   a. to limit bleeding after a surgical wound
   b. to cover a "black eye"
   c. to limit bacteria from reaching the eye
   d. to immobilize the eyelids to promote corneal epithelial healing

ANSWER   **b.** to cover a "black eye"

EXPLANATION   By putting pressure on the eye, the patch can control a tendency for the eye to bleed. The occlusive nature of the patch prevents outside bacteria from reaching the eye, limiting the chances for infection. With the eyelids immobilized, the abrasive effect of the lids blinking over a corneal epithelial defect is eliminated, helping the defect to heal. These are all medical reasons for a pressure patch. Although a patch might hide bruising of the eyelids ("black eye"), this is a cosmetic issue and not a reason for patching. (Newmark 2006, 254)

54   What is the first step in using a manual lensmeter to determine the power of an eyeglass lens?

   a. Correctly position the eyeglasses in the lensmeter.
   b. Turn the power drum to a high minus position.
   c. Turn the power drum to a high plus position.
   d. Focus the eyepiece of the lensmeter.

ANSWER   **d.** Focus the eyepiece of the lensmeter.

EXPLANATION   Always check the focus of the eyepiece before using a manual lensmeter. If you do not have the eyepiece in focus, your readings of the eyeglass power may be incorrect. Correct positioning of the eyeglasses and operation of the power drum are further steps in determining the lens power of the eyeglasses. (Newmark 2006, 71)

55   What change must be made on the lensmeter to be able to read a cylinder lens that is in the plus convention into the minus format?

   a. Change the axis 180°.
   b. Change the axis 45°.
   c. Change the axis 90°.
   d. Change the axis to zero.

ANSWER   **c.** Change the axis 90°.

EXPLANATION   The plus cylinder convention is always 90°opposite to the minus format and vice versa. Changing the cylinder convention will also alter the sphere power. What happens in the lensmeter is basically what is happening when one carries out a transposition of a lens prescription on paper from plus to minus cylinder. An example of the same prescription in the two conventions follows: –1.50 + 0.50 × 060 plus cylinder and –1.00 –0.50 × 150 minus cylinder. (Newmark 2006, 71–72)

56   The following occurs while taking a lensmeter reading: the single lines focus at –2.50; the triple lines focus at –1.00 with the axis at 085°. What would be the eyeglass prescription?

   a. –2.50 –1.00 axis 175
   b. –2.50 +1.50 axis 085
   c. –1.00 –2.50 axis 175
   d. –3.50 –1.00 axis 085

ANSWER   **b.** –2.50 +1.50 axis 085

EXPLANATION   The single lines focused at –2.50, so the sphere power is –2.50. The triple lines focused at –1.00; hence 1.50 less was needed from the –2.50 sphere to focus on the cylinder power. The axis read 085° on the cylinder axis wheel, so that is the axis for the +1.50 cylinder. All the other prescriptions are incorrect because in plus cylinder lensmeter readings the single lines focus at the sphere power (–2.50) and the triple lines focus on the cylinder (–1.00) only when the axis is set correctly on the cylinder axis wheel (in this case 085). The only calculation required is to determine the prescription cylinder power which, in this case, is 1.50 less minus (or +1.50) then the sphere power (–2.50). (Newmark 2006, 71)

57   What is the best test to document the shape and average number of corneal endothelial cells in a patient with Fuchs corneal dystrophy?

   a. fundus photography
   b. external photography
   c. slit-lamp photography
   d. specular microscopy photography

ANSWER   **d.** specular microscopy photography

EXPLANATION   Specular microscopy is a test of the corneal endothelium that allows one to determine the average number of endothelial cells present in the central cornea (figure). The photograph that is obtained with this test also allows the ophthalmologist to determine the size and geometric shape of the endothelial cells. Fundus photography images the retina and optic disc. External photography images the eye's outer structures. Slit-lamp photography images the anterior structures of the globe. (Newmark 2006, 145)

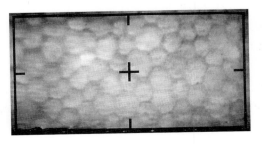

Specular photograph showing normal endothelial cells. (Reproduced, with permission, from Newmark E, ed. *Ophthalmic Medical Assisting: An Independent Study Course*, 4th ed. San Francisco: American Academy of Ophthalmology; 2006.)

58   When an ophthalmologist orders a photographic test to document the position of the eyelid in a patient with ptosis, what type of ophthalmic photography is indicated?

a. fundus photography
b. external photography
c. slit-lamp photography
d. specular microscopy photography

ANSWER   **b.** external photography

EXPLANATION   Position of the eyelid and any lesion of the face, eyelid, or ocular adnexa depend upon external photography. Fundus photography images the retina and optic disc. Slit-lamp photography images the anterior structures of the globe. Specular microscopy photography images the corneal endothelium. (Newmark 2006, 145)

59   The figure shows an example of what type of ophthalmic test?

a. specular microscopy
b. slit-lamp photography
c. fundus photography
d. slit-lamp gonioscopic photography

ANSWER   **b.** slit-lamp photography

EXPLANATION   The slit beam is angled to provide an appreciation of the depth of the anterior chamber. The broad beam on the right of the image is on the more-anterior part of the cornea, while the more-narrow beam on the left falls on the anterior iris and lens surface. The white spot on the anterior lens surface is a polar cataract. The area in between these 2 beams is the anterior chamber. Specular microscopy images the endothelial layer of the cornea. Fundus photography images the retina and optic disc. Slit-lamp gonioscopic photography images the anterior chamber angle structures. (Newmark 2006, 146)

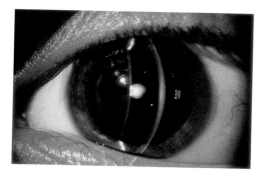

Slit-lamp photography. (Reproduced, with permission, from Rosenfeld SI, *Basic and Clinical Science Course*, Section 11: Lens and Cataract, American Academy of Ophthalmology, 2004–2005.)

60   What ophthalmic photographic test uses the techniques of sclerotic scatter and retroillumination to evaluate the cornea and media opacities?

a. fundus photography
b. external photography

  c. slit-lamp photography

  d. specular microscopy photography

ANSWER **c.** slit-lamp photography

EXPLANATION Sclerotic scatter and retroillumination are techniques used with slit-lamp photography (figure) to highlight features of the cornea and media opacities. This indirect form of illumination of the cornea allows corneal opacities and guttata to be evaluated in a manner that is often superior to direct illumination of the opacity itself. Fundus photography images the retina and optic disc. External photography images the eye's outer structures. Specular microscopy photography images the corneal endothelium. (Newmark 2006, 145–146)

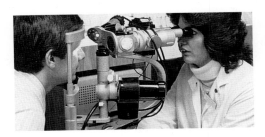

Slit-lamp photography of the anterior segment of the eye. (Reproduced, with permission, from Newmark E, ed. *Ophthalmic Medical Assisting: An Independent Study Course,* 4th ed. San Francisco: American Academy of Ophthalmology; 2006.)

61 How do optical coherence tomography (OCT), GDx scanning laser polarimetry with variable corneal compensation, and the Heidelberg retinal tomograph allow the ophthalmologist to interpret the 3-dimensional depiction of the optic nerve and retinal nerve fiber layer in glaucoma patients?

  a. by comparison with a database of age-matched "normal" patients

  b. by comparison with a database of other patients with glaucoma

  c. by comparison with a database of other age-matched patients with glaucoma

  d. by comparison with a database of "normal" patients

ANSWER **a.** by comparison with a database of age-matched "normal" patients

EXPLANATION These tests rely upon normative databases to compare the results from the patient of interest to age-matched "normal" patients. This helps the ophthalmologist determine how far away from "normal" the patient of interest appears to be. (Newmark 2006, 147)

62 What test is used to measure the axial length of the globe in preparation for intraocular lens calculations for patients about to undergo cataract surgery?

  a. B-scan (B-mode) ultrasonography

  b. 3-dimensional ultrasonography

  c. A-scan (A-mode) ultrasonography

  d. optical coherence tomography

ANSWER **c.** A-scan (A-mode) ultrasonography

EXPLANATION   A-scan ultrasonography uses sound waves traveling in a straight line to measure the distance between the front of the cornea and the front of the retina to determine the axial length of the eye. This distance, expressed in millimeters, is used to calculate the power of the intraocular lens to be used for a patient about to undergo cataract surgery. B-scan is used to image the intraocular and periocular structures. 3-D ultrasonography adds a third dimension to B-scan images. Optical coherence tomography images the thickness of the retinal nerve fiber layer and thickness of the central retina. (Newmark 2006, 147)

63   Patients with what type of allergy should not undergo intravenous indocyanine green (ICG) fundus angiography?

a. peanuts
b. penicillin
c. morphine
d. shellfish

ANSWER   d. shellfish

EXPLANATION   Fundus angiography makes it possible to view detail in retinal blood vessels of the eye after a dye solution has been injected into a vein in the patient's arm. Indocyanine green dye should be avoided in patients with an allergy to shellfish. Patients with an iodine allergy should also avoid intravenous ICG fundus angiography. (Newmark 2006, 147)

64   What is the focal length of a spectacle lens with a power of +5.00 diopters?

a. 0.50 meters
b. 5.00 meters
c. 2.00 meters
d. 0.20 meters

ANSWER   d. 0.20 meters

EXPLANATION   The focal length is inversely related to the power of the lens. This means that the stronger the lens power, the shorter the focal length. In mathematical terms, the power of a lens is equal to the reciprocal of the focal length measured in meters. It is expressed as the formula $D = 1/F$, where D = diopters (power of the lens) and F = the focal length in meters. (Newmark 2006, 57)

65   What type of lens best corrects hyperopia with astigmatism?

a. prism
b. cylindrical lens
c. spherical lens
d. spherocylindrical lens

ANSWER   d. spherocylindrical lens

EXPLANATION   The basic types of ophthalmic lenses used to test for and correct refractive errors are spheres, cylinders, and a combination of both. Spherocylinder lenses are best for correcting a combination of a spherical and astigmatic error. (Newmark 2006, 62)

66   If a ray of light traveling through a lens is deviated 1 centimeter at 1 meter of distance, what is the power of the lens?

    a. 1 diopter of myopia
    b. 1 diopter of astigmatism
    c. 1 prism diopter
    d. 1 diopter of add

ANSWER   **c.** 1 prism diopter

EXPLANATION   Because of its shape, a prism deviates (refracts) light rays toward its base. This effect causes objects viewed through prisms to appear displaced toward the prism apex. One prism diopter (1 PD) deviates parallel rays of light 1 centimeter at a distance of 100 centimeters or 1 meter. (Newmark 2006, 62)

67   During retinoscopy, what type of light reflex is seen in a myopic eye?

    a. moves in the same direction as the streak of light
    b. moves in the opposite direction as the streak of light
    c. does not appear to have any movement
    d. streak of light has a red glow

ANSWER   **b.** moves in the opposite direction as the streak of light

EXPLANATION   Retinoscopy is an objective method that uses a streak of light to determine the patient's approximate refraction. As the examiner watches the light sweep across the pupil, different refractive errors produce characteristic movements of the reflex that appears. For a myopic patient, an against-motion light reflex will occur (the reflex moves in the opposite direction from the streak). If a patient is hyperopic, a with-motion light reflex will occur. When the true prescription is determined and the vision is neutralized, there will be no apparent reflex movement or a red glow is seen in the pupil. (Newmark 2006, 64–65)

68   An automated objective refractor is helpful in what tasks?

    a. making an estimate of the prescription for eyeglasses
    b. refining a subjective refraction
    c. determining the refractive error in a patient with moderate cataracts
    d. measuring the refractive error in a patient with very small pupils

ANSWER   **a.** making an estimate of the prescription for eyeglasses

EXPLANATION   An automated objective refractor estimates the prescription that may be needed for eyeglasses, but the prescription must then be refined with a phoropter or with trial lenses in a trial frame. Automated objective refractors may be less accurate in patients with very small pupils and in patients with cataracts. (Newmark 2006, 68)

69   A cross cylinder may be used to refine the refractive error correction of eyes with what condition?

a. diplopia
b. astigmatism
c. presbyopia
d. hypermetropia

ANSWER   b. astigmatism

EXPLANATION   A cross cylinder is used to refine both the cylindrical power and the cylindrical axis needed to correct astigmatism. Prisms are used to refine the prismatic power needed to correct diplopia. Plus (converging) lenses are used to refine the refractive error needed to correct presbyopia and hypermetropia (hyperopia). (Newmark 2006, 66–67)

70   In tightening or replacing a screw on an eyeglass frame, a droplet of what substance should be used to secure the screw?

a. epoxy resin
b. white glue
c. shellac
d. clear fingernail polish

ANSWER   d. clear fingernail polish

EXPLANATION   A tiny thing can sometimes be a major annoyance, and an eyeglass screw is a good example. Clear fingernail polish is inexpensive, easy to use, and decreases the chance of the tightened screw to back out. Epoxy resin will not allow the screw to be removed if the glasses need future repair. Shellac will hold the screw, but shellac is more difficult to obtain, to maintain, and to apply. White glue will not hold the screw. (Newmark 2006, 187)

71   How can light transmission through an eyeglass lens be increased?

a. applying an antireflective coating onto the lens
b. tinting the lens a light yellow color
c. increasing the size of the lens
d. placing a high polish on both the front and back surfaces of the lens

ANSWER   a. applying an antireflective coating onto the lens

EXPLANATION   Antireflective coatings slightly increase the light transmission through eyeglass lenses from about 90% to 95% or more, although most patients do not notice this increase. A light yellow tint, a larger lens, and polished surfaces do not improve light transmission of a lens. (Newmark 2006, 179–180)

72   What is the base curve of an eyeglass lens?

    a. the curve on the front surface of the lens
    b. the curve on the back surface of the lens
    c. the smaller of the front and back surface curves
    d. the larger of the front and back surface curves

ANSWER   **a.** the curve on the front surface of the lens

EXPLANATION   If the base curves of eyeglass lenses are changed from those that a patient has comfortably worn in his or her old eyeglasses, he or she may experience eyestrain or discomfort with the new eyeglasses. The base curve is always defined as the spherical curve of the distance correction on the front surface of the eyeglass lens. For an accurate measurement with a Geneva lens gauge, be careful not to place the contacts of the lens gauge on the bifocal or the progressive addition portion of a multifocal lens. The old definition of base curve used the back surface curve of the lens. Today that definition has been abandoned. (Newmark 2006, 184–185)

73   What is the size of the area applanated on the cornea by the Goldmann tonometer?

    a. 1 square millimeter
    b. 3.06 square millimeters
    c. 10 square millimeters
    d. irrelevant to the measurement

ANSWER   **b.** 3.06 square millimeters

EXPLANATION   The size of the applanated (flattened) area of the cornea is fixed by the size of the tonometer tip. For the Goldmann tonometer, it is 3.06 square millimeters. (Newmark 2006, 129)

74   What statement applies to a patient with an intraocular pressure reading of 25 mm Hg on Goldmann applanation tonometry?

    a. definitely has glaucoma
    b. definitely does not have glaucoma
    c. may actually have lower intraocular pressure
    d. should be rechecked 1 hour later

ANSWER   **c.** may actually have lower intraocular pressure

EXPLANATION   The pressure reading may be overestimated, depending upon the central corneal thickness. An isolated pressure reading cannot rule out or confirm glaucoma. If the pressure is to be rechecked, it should be done immediately; waiting 1 hour accomplishes nothing. (Newmark 2006, 126–132)

75   The tip of the Goldmann tonometer is round, yet the mires seen during applanation tonometry appear as 2 semicircles. How is this achieved?

    a. the use of a prism within the tip
    b. the optics of the cornea itself
    c. the use of a high plus lens
    d. an artifact of a circular object touching the cornea

ANSWER   **a.** the use of a prism within the tip

EXPLANATION   The split circle appearance of the mires is achieved by a prism. (Newmark 2006, 129–130)

76   Which of the following methods might be the most accurate for measuring intraocular pressure in an eye with a scarred, irregular cornea?

    a. Goldmann tonometry
    b. palpation
    c. air-puff tonometry
    d. Tono-Pen

ANSWER   **d.** Tono-Pen

EXPLANATION   The Tono-Pen provides the most accurate measurement of the intraocular pressure when faced with a scarred or irregular cornea. Palpation gives only a rough estimate of intraocular pressure and is not very accurate. Goldmann (applanation) and air-puff tonometers will not give accurate readings when the cornea is irregular. (Newmark 2006, 129–130; Wilson 2009)

77   Of the following, what is the accurate second part of the phrase, "The higher the scale reading on the Schiøtz tonometer ... "?

    a. the higher the intraocular pressure
    b. the lower the intraocular pressure
    c. the less the cornea has been indented
    d. the more resistance to compression

ANSWER   **b.** the lower the intraocular pressure

EXPLANATION   The Schiøtz tonometer measures intraocular pressure by applying a weight to the cornea. The scale on the instrument reflects how much the cornea has been indented by the weight; the higher the number, the more the indentation, corresponding to lower intraocular pressure (ie, less intraocular force pushing back on the instrument; the less the cornea resists compression). (Newmark 2006, 131)

78   What is the derivation of the word *laser*?

    a. light amplified by sensory emission of radiation
    b. light amplification by stimulated emission of radiation

      c. light amplitude synonymous with emitted radiation

      d. longitudinal aberrations of seismographic emitted radio waves

ANSWER   **b.** light amplification by stimulated emission of radiation

EXPLANATION   Lasers are a source of an extremely intense form of monochromatic light organized in a concentrated beam that can cut, burn, disrupt, destroy, alter, or vaporize tissue. The word *laser* is an acronym for **L**ight **A**mplification by **S**timulated **E**mission of **R**adiation. (Newmark 2006, 296)

79   Which phrase applies to aseptic technique?

      a. is usually not necessary in an office procedure

      b. limited to sterilizing instruments and wearing gloves

      c. is important because it reduces the risk of infection

      d. is only required in a hospital

ANSWER   **c.** is important because it reduces the risk of infection

EXPLANATION   Aseptic technique is employed in office and hospital surgeries. It is designed to maintain a sterile surgical environment in order to limit the risk of infection. In an office setting aseptic technique consists of several components: using sterile instruments and supplies; preparing the patient's operative site with germicidal solutions (prepping); performing a surgical scrub and putting on sterile gloves; and maintaining sterility and preventing contamination. (Newmark 2006, 255)

80   The ophthalmic medical assistant's duties related to surgery include which of the following?

      a. getting the patient's consent

      b. sterilizing the instruments

      c. filling out the encounter form

      d. talking to the patient's family

ANSWER   **b.** sterilizing the instruments

EXPLANATION   The ophthalmic surgical assistant's responsibilities for minor surgery include sterilizing the instruments. In addition, the surgical assistant has the following responsibilities: ensure asepsis of the surgical area; prepare the patient for surgery; prepare the instrument tray; assist the surgeon during the procedure; and clean and dispose of instruments and materials after surgery.

Informed consent is a process, not simply a signed form. The assistant may obtain the signature, but the discussion of the details of the procedure and the risk and benefits must be between the doctor and patient. It is the doctor's responsibility to fill out the encounter form correctly, as the doctor is subject to insurance laws for correct coding. The physician should talk to the family following the procedure to discuss the outcome and postoperative care of the patient. (Newmark 2006, 244–245, 255)

81   What is the most common opacity affecting the ocular media?

  a. cataract
  b. vitreous hemorrhage
  c. glaucoma
  d. scotoma

ANSWER   **a.** cataract

EXPLANATION   A cataract is an opacity in the lens and is the most common abnormality affecting the ocular media. A vitreous hemorrhage is also an opacity in the ocular media, but clinically it is infrequently seen. Glaucoma is an ocular disease that affects the optic nerve. A scotoma is a visual field defect. (Newmark 2006, 20, 142)

82   If the patient cannot see the big "E" (20/400) on the Snellen acuity chart when best corrected, what does this indicate?

  a. The patient is blind.
  b. The patient should have cataract surgery.
  c. The patient should be tested for count fingers (CF), hand motions (HM), or light perception (LP) vision.
  d. The patient has a constricted visual field.

ANSWER   **c.** The patient should be tested for count fingers (CF), hand motions (HM), or light perception (LP) vision.

EXPLANATION   Patients with less than 20/400 vision are not necessarily blind nor have a constricted peripheral visual field. They should be tested for low vision with CF, HM, or LP vision tests. The need for cataract surgery cannot be determined solely by a visual acuity measurement. (Newmark 2006, 231)

83   Which phrase applies to the super pinhole test?

  a. measures current vision after a refraction
  b. requires a dilated pupil
  c. can be performed regardless of the capability of the patient
  d. is rarely helpful

ANSWER   **b.** requires a dilated pupil

EXPLANATION   Through a dilated pupil, looking through an opaque occluder with pinholes held before the eye (figure), a capable patient can often find a window in his or her ocular opacity, thereby frequently allowing the approximate prediction of postoperative vision. Patients with sharp awareness seem to be better candidates for this test. (Newmark 2006, 142)

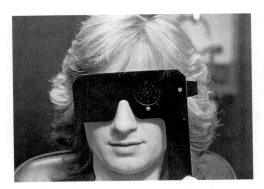

An opaque occluder with pinholes covers the dilated left eye. The patient views the eye chart through one of the pinholes. (Reproduced, with permission, from Newmark E, ed. *Ophthalmic Medical Assisting: An Independent Study Course*, 4th ed. San Francisco: American Academy of Ophthalmology, 2006.)

84   Which statement is correct regarding visual acuity testing in the pediatric patient?

   a. Visual acuity cannot be assessed for the preliterate child.
   b. A papoose board is routinely used for infants.
   c. The examination method is not different than for adults.
   d. A principle goal is to assess visual acuity without intimidating the child.

ANSWER   **d.** A principle goal is to assess visual acuity without intimidating the child.

EXPLANATION   Visual acuity can be assessed in the pediatric patient. Several strategies are used to assess vision in the preliterate child. A papoose board may occasionally be used to immobilize an infant for some examination needs but is not used for visual assessment. Both history taking and examination methods are different for children than for adults. (Newmark 2006, 233–235)

85   What does the pinhole acuity test measure?

   a. the patient's corrected vision with a proper refraction
   b. the best vision the patient would be expected to achieve if the media were clear
   c. the patient's ability to read
   d. the patient's vision with both eyes looking through pinholes

ANSWER   **a.** the patient's corrected vision with a proper refraction

EXPLANATION   In the pinhole acuity test, the patient views the Snellen acuity chart through a pinhole occluder. The pinhole allows only parallel rays of light to enter the eye and so approximates the vision achieved with a proper refraction. Opacities in the media decrease the best-corrected vision and so decrease the pinhole vision as well. The test must be performed with 1 eye at a time, fully occluding the opposite eye. The ability to read is a cerebral function and is not measured by pinhole vision. (Newmark 2006, 119)

86   Visual potential tests include which of the following?

   a. testing for near vision
   b. refracting the patient after dilation
   c. PAM, interferometer, and super pinhole
   d. visual field

ANSWER   **c.** PAM, interferometer, and super pinhole

EXPLANATION   Testing for near vision and a refraction determine current vision, which will be decreased by the effect of any opacities in the ocular media. The potential acuity meter (PAM), interferometer, and super pinhole seek to bypass opacities in the media and are used to predict the potential vision after the opacity is removed. A visual field is not a measurement of potential visual acuity. (Newmark 2006, 142–143)

87   A patient complains of transient shimmering vision that affected the right half of the visual field in each eye. The shimmering vision lasted about 20 minutes and resolved completely. The diagnosis is ophthalmic migraine (migraine without the headache). Which part of the brain was affected by the transient blood vessel spasm?

    a. the right occipital area
    b. the left occipital area
    c. the right frontal cortex
    d. the left frontal cortex

ANSWER   **b.** the left occipital area

EXPLANATION   A transient change in blood flow can affect the area of the brain responsible for vision. The scenario described represents a right hemianopic defect due to a vascular spasm on the left side of the brain. The frontal cortex does not contain any of the fibers of the visual pathway (figure), and a migraine arising there would not affect the visual field. (Newmark 2006, 154, 167)

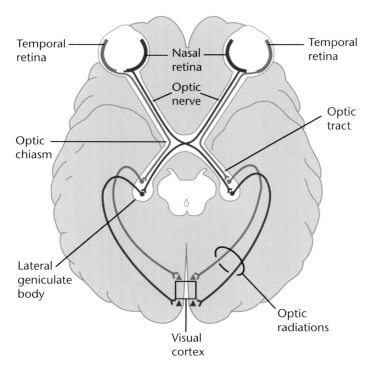

The visual pathway. (Reproduced, with permission, from Newmark E, ed. *Ophthalmic Medical Assisting: An Independent Study Course,* 4th ed. San Francisco: American Academy of Ophthalmology, 2006.)

88   Where anatomically do the optic nerve fibers come together and reorganize?

　　a. optical center
　　b. optic chiasm
　　c. fovea
　　d. visual pathway

ANSWER   **b.** optic chiasm

EXPLANATION   The optic nerve fibers from both eyes extend posteriorly from the orbits and come together near the center of the skull in a structure called the optic chiasm. In the optic chiasm the fibers from the nasal retina in both eyes cross to the opposite side of the brain. The temporal fibers of the retina in both eyes remain on the original side. The chiasm is the only place where the optic nerve fibers come together to reorganize. The optical center is the single point of a lens that provides optimal vision. The fovea is the center of the macula that allows for the clearest central vision. The visual pathway is the route the neurons follow from the eyeball to the visual cortex of the brain. (Newmark 2006, 154)

89   The Humphrey computerized perimeter is an automated system for measuring a patient's visual field. How are test points presented?

　　a. kinetic strategy
　　b. static testing
　　c. contrast sensitivity
　　d. object size differences

ANSWER   **b.** static testing

EXPLANATION   Automated devices such as the Humphrey visual field perimeter use static testing for presenting test points. The target is a given size, and the instrument increases the brightness until the patient sees it. Kinetic testing is used in the Goldmann visual field perimeter in which the examiner brings a moving target into the normal boundaries of the field of vision until the patient sees it. Contrast sensitivity tests the ability to distinguish between light and dark areas, useful in the diagnosis of cataracts and is not a perimeter. (Newmark 2006, 161)

90   What is the term for an abnormal visual field that is missing the right or left quadrant?

　　a. Bjerrum scotoma
　　b. hemianopia
　　c. quadrantanopia
　　d. normal visual field

ANSWER   **c.** quadrantanopia

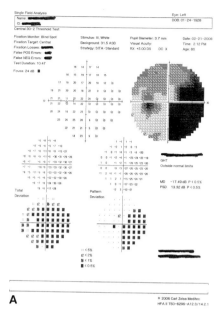
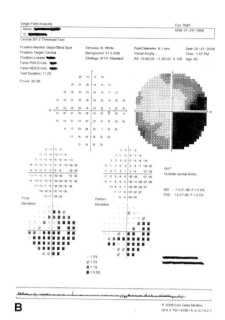

Quadrantanopia. A. Left eye. B. Right eye.

EXPLANATION   A quadrantanopia (figure) is the loss of the right or left upper or lower quarter of the visual field respecting the vertical nerve fiber boundary. A Bjerrum scotoma is a visual field defect that starts at or near the physiologic blind spot and spreads nasally as a gradually widening band. A hemianopia is loss of half the visual field. A normal visual field has no areas of loss, except the blind spot caused by the optic nerve. (Newmark 2006, 166)

91   When performing a visual field test, if the pupil is smaller than 2 mm, what should you do?

a. Continue with the test.
b. Request permission to dilate the pupil.
c. Use a more powerful lens.
d. Perform the visual field test twice.

ANSWER   **b.** Request permission to dilate the pupil.

EXPLANATION   Ask permission to dilate the pupil. With a pupil 2 mm or smaller, the sensitivity to the test is markedly reduced. If you continue with the test, it will be less accurate due to different properties of light and how it passes through a small pupil. A more powerful lens will not help improve detecting light but rather make the focus wrong. Repeating the test will likely give the same inaccurate results as the problem is how light passes through a pupil. (Newmark 2006, 171)

92   During perimetry, what is the usual reason for taping the upper eyelid to keep it out of the field of view?

a. provides a break for restless patients

b. increases the amount of light captured by the eye
c. improves the test results if the patient has astigmatism
d. improves the test results if the patient has ptosis

ANSWER   **d.** improves the test results if the patient has ptosis

EXPLANATION   Taping the upper eyelid of a patient with ptosis uncovers the superior visual field, allowing the patient to perform much better on the test. The taped upper eyelid test is often used to justify noncosmetic repair of ptosis. Perimetry should be performed in a single session when possible to avoid changes in light adaptation, which confound the results. Taping the upper eyelid does not increase the amount of light that enters the eye for any test spots within the region of perception. Taping has no effect on astigmatism. (Newmark 2006, 171)

93   An elderly patient with no past eye or medical problems presents with nausea, sudden onset of right eye pain, and blurred vision with haloes around lights. What is the likely explanation?

a. mature cataract
b. corneal ulcer
c. endophthalmitis
d. acute angle-closure glaucoma

ANSWER   **d.** acute angle-closure glaucoma

EXPLANATION   Acute angle-closure glaucoma generally occurs in an older patient and causes the symptoms described. It is a true ophthalmic emergency. A mature cataract does not cause sudden loss of vision and, by itself, is not a cause of pain. A corneal ulcer may cause these symptoms, but it typically occurs as a complication of contact lens wear, trauma, or in an eye with previous corneal disease. Endophthalmitis is a complication of past eye surgery, ocular trauma, or in a patient with significant medical problems. (Newmark 2006, 37)

94   What function does the Farnsworth-Munsell D-15 test have in office practice?

a. tests color vision
b. measures central retinal thickness
c. measures corneal curvature
d. tests distance visual acuity

ANSWER   **a.** tests color vision

EXPLANATION   The Farnsworth-Munsell D-15 test, also called the *15-hue test*, is a specialized test of color vision. In this test, 15 pastel-colored chips of similar brightness must be arranged by the patient in a specific color sequence (figure). Patients with normal color vision have no trouble with the test, but people with color vision deficiencies will often make characteristic mistakes. Optical coherence tomography (OCT) measures central retinal thickness. Corneal curvature is measured by a keratometer or by corneal topography. Tests of distance visual acuity employ a Snellen acuity chart. (Newmark 2006, 135–136)

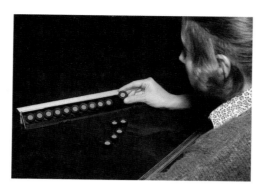

The 15-hue test of color vision. (Reproduced, with permission, from Newmark E, ed. *Ophthalmic Medical Assisting: An Independent Study Course,* 4th ed. San Francisco: American Academy of Ophthalmology; 2006.)

95   Glare testing is most useful in the evaluation of which of the following?

    a. cataract
    b. glaucoma
    c. macular degeneration
    d. uveitis

ANSWER   **a.** cataract

EXPLANATION   Glare testing is a method of determining how much visual acuity is affected due to a cataract. Glaucoma is evaluated by intraocular pressure, optic disc, and visual field studies. Macular degeneration is evaluated by visual assessment, Amsler grid, and fundus examination. Uveitis is evaluated by slit-lamp exam. (Newmark 2006, 143)

96   If the axial length of the eye measured is shorter than the actual axial length, how will the postoperative refraction be affected?

    a. no effect
    b. more hyperopia than anticipated
    c. more myopia than anticipated
    d. more astigmatism than anticipated

ANSWER   **c.** more myopia than anticipated

EXPLANATION   If the axial length measured is shorter than the actual axial length, the patient's eye will seem more hyperopic than it actually is. In addition, the incorrect measurement will increase the plus power of the intraocular lens calculation, which will leave the patient myopic postoperatively. (Newmark 2006, 147–148)

97   A patient has an axial length of 26.00 mm and K readings of 44.00 D. Which of the following statements is true?

    a. This is average, and the patient will have no significant refractive error.
    b. This is a short eye with flat curvature, and the patient will be hyperopic.
    c. This is a long eye with flat curvature, and the patient will be myopic.
    d. This is a long eye with steep curvature, and the patient will be myopic.

ANSWER   **d.** This is a long eye with steep curvature, and the patient will be myopic.

EXPLANATION   An axial length of 26 mm is longer than average (23.50) and corneal curvature of 44.00 D is steeper than average (43.00). A longer eye and steeper cornea make the eye more myopic; therefore, the image of an object focuses in front of the retina. (Kendall 1991, 161–162)

98   Evaluation of color vision is often performed using which of the following?

    a. direct ophthalmoscope
    b. pseudoisochromatic test plates
    c. Schirmer test
    d. Worth four-dot test

ANSWER   **b.** pseudoisochromatic test plates

EXPLANATION   Pseudoisochromatic test plates (figure) are used to check for color vision abnormalities and consist of patterns of colored and gray dots. The direct ophthalmoscope is used primarily to view intraocular structures, including the optic disc and central retina. Schirmer testing is used to evaluate tear secretion. The Worth four-dot test is designed to show whether a patient is using both eyes together. (Newmark 2006, 135–136)

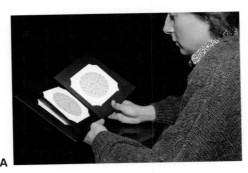

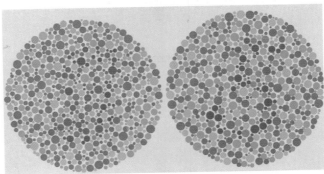

(A) Pseudoisochromatic color plates used to test color vision. The patient must detect numbers or figures embedded in an array of colored dots. (B) Pseudoisochromatic color plates in greater detail. (Part A reproduced, with permission, from Newmark E, ed. *Ophthalmic Medical Assisting: An Independent Study Course*, 4th ed. San Francisco: American Academy of Ophthalmology; 2006. Part B reproduced, with permission, from Regillo C, *Basic and Clinical Science Course*, Section 12: Retina and Vitreous. San Francisco: American Academy of Ophthalmology; 2004.)

99   A patient has increased corneal thickness. What problem may arise when this patient's intraocular pressure (IOP) is measured with an applanation tonometer?

  a. A higher concentration of anesthetic is necessary to numb the cornea.
  b. The mires (prism image) will be distorted and irregular.
  c. The IOP reading will be falsely low.
  d. The IOP reading will be falsely high.

ANSWER   d. The IOP reading will be falsely high.

EXPLANATION   The Goldmann applanation tonometer is designed with the assumption that the cornea is of average thickness. The instrument measures the pressure necessary to flatten a fixed area of the cornea. A thicker cornea creates more resistance to this flattening, causing a falsely high pressure reading. A thinner cornea offers less resistance to flattening, yielding a falsely low pressure reading. This may explain why some patients who never show a pressure over 20 mm Hg have glaucomatous optic nerve damage. Corneal thickness should be measured in patients suspected of having glaucoma to avoid making false assumptions based on incorrect IOP measurements. Higher concentrations of anesthetic are not required for applanation tonometry under any circumstances. Distorted mires occur with irregular corneal surfaces but not with otherwise normal thinner or thicker corneas. (Newmark 2006, 36; Stein 2006, 453)

100   If the anterior chamber is shallow, the flashlight test will show which of the following?

  a. The iris is evenly illuminated.
  b. The iris is shadowed on the temporal side.
  c. The iris is shadowed on the nasal side.
  d. The pupil is unable to constrict normally.

ANSWER   c. The iris is shadowed on the nasal side.

EXPLANATION   When the flashlight is shined from the temporal limbus, across the iris, the iris should be evenly illuminated if the anterior chamber is deep. If the anterior chamber is shallow, there will be shadowing of the nasal side of the iris. (Newmark 2006, 133)

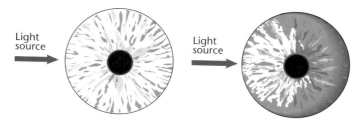

Performing the flashlight test to estimate anterior depth. Left: In an eye with a normally shaped anterior chamber and iris, the nasal half of the iris will be illuminated like the temporal half. Right: In an eye with a shallow anterior chamber and narrow chamber angle, about two-thirds of the nasal portion of the iris will appear in shadow. (Reproduced, with permission, from Newmark E, ed. *Ophthalmic Medical Assisting: An Independent Study Course*, 4th ed. San Francisco: American Academy of Ophthalmology; 2006.)

Certified Ophthalmic Assistant Exam Study Guide

Practice Test Answer Key

Use this answer key to score the answers you recorded on the *Practice Test Answer Sheet* in the back of Section Three.

1	d	26	c	51	c	76	d
2	a	27	d	52	b	77	b
3	b	28	a	53	b	78	b
4	b	29	a	54	d	79	c
5	a	30	a	55	c	80	b
6	b	31	c	56	b	81	a
7	a	32	d	57	d	82	c
8	c	33	c	58	b	83	b
9	c	34	a	59	b	84	d
10	c	35	b	60	c	85	a
11	b	36	a	61	a	86	c
12	c	37	c	62	c	87	b
13	d	38	c	63	d	88	b
14	a	39	c	64	d	89	b
15	b	40	a	65	d	90	c
16	c	41	d	66	c	91	b
17	a	42	d	67	b	92	d
18	c	43	d	68	a	93	d
19	a	44	c	69	b	94	a
20	c	45	a	70	d	95	a
21	a	46	c	71	a	96	c
22	b	47	d	72	a	97	d
23	c	48	b	73	b	98	b
24	d	49	a	74	c	99	d
25	b	50	a	75	a	100	c

Suggested Reading

American Academy of Ophthalmology. *Minimizing Transmission of Bloodborne Pathogens and Surface Infectious Agents in Ophthalmic Offices and Operating Rooms.* Clinical Statement. San Francisco: American Academy of Ophthalmology; 2002.

Bradford C, ed. *Basic Ophthalmology*, 8th ed. San Francisco: American Academy of Ophthalmology, 2004.

Centers for Disease Control and Prevention. Infection control guidelines. Web page of documents related to infection control. http://www.cdc.gov/ncidod/dhqp/guidelines.html [accessed February 1, 2010].

JCAHPO. Criteria for certification and recertification for ophthalmic medical personnel. http://www.jcahpo.org/certification/pdfs/CriteriaforCert_FULL.pdf [accessed February 1, 2010].

Kendall CJ. *Ophthalmic Echography.* Ophthalmic Technical Skills Series. Thorofare, NJ: Slack, 1991.

Ledford JK, Sanders VN. *The Slit-Lamp Primer.* 2nd ed. Thorofare, NJ: Slack, 2006:18.

Newmark E, ed. *Ophthalmic Medical Assisting: An Independent Study Course*, 4th ed. San Francisco: American Academy of Ophthalmology, 2006.

Niffenegger JH, Scrimo S. Fluorescein angiography: basic principles. *Refinements.* 2000;4(1):2–3.

Patel S, Blades KJ. *The Dry Eye: A Practical Approach.* Oxford, UK: Butterworth-Heinemann, 2003.

Shetlar DM, Chair. Other histologic changes in diabetes. In: *Ophthalmic Pathology.* Basic and Clinical Science Course, Section 4. San Francisco: American Academy of Ophthalmology, 2008–2009.

Stein HA, Stein RM, Freeman MI. *The Ophthalmic Assistant: A Text for Allied and Associated Ophthalmic Personnel*, 8th ed. St Louis: Mosby, 2006.

Trobe JD. *The Physician's Guide to Eye Care*, 3rd ed. San Francisco: American Academy of Ophthalmology, 2006.

Waldron RG. B-scan ultrasound: indications and applications. *Refinements.* 1999; 3(1):1–14.

Wilson FM, ed. *Practical Ophthalmology*, 6th ed. San Francisco: American Academy of Ophthalmology, 2009.

Index